An Introduction to Nursing

Sheila Collins
Edith Parker

with contributions from

Barbara McNulty
Jennifer Raiman
Veronica Chapman
Jill Macleod Clark
Stephen Kirkham
Daphne Hill

MACMILLAN

First published 1983
Reprinted (with corrections) 1984

Published by
MACMILLAN EDUCATION LTD
Houndmills, Basingstoke, Hampshire RG21 2XS
and London
Associated companies in Auckland, Delhi, Dublin,
Gaborone, Hamburg, Harare, Hong Kong,
Johannesburg, Kuala Lumpur, Lagos, Manzini,
Melbourne, Mexico City, Nairobi, New York,
Singapore and Tokyo

ISBN 0 333 35468 0 (hard cover)
      0 333 35207 6 (paper cover)
      0 333 35826 0 (paper cover set)

Printed in England by
Pindar Print Limited, Scarborough, North Yorkshire.

5.50

An Introduction to Nursing

The Contributors

Barbara J. McNulty, SRN, SCM, FRCN, works in Wales as a counsellor with particular concern for the bereaved. Her interest in the problems of families caring for dying patients at home, and the needs of those patients, led her to joining St Christopher's Hospice in 1967 when it first opened, and here she pioneered and developed the Home Care Service. She has written several articles on death and bereavement for American and British nursing journals.

Jennifer Raiman, SRN, is a Research Associate at the Department of Pharmacology and Therapeutics at The London Hospital, and is currently undertaking research into pain. She teaches nurses and medical students about the care of the dying and pain control. She has also trained and worked as a marriage guidance counsellor.

Veronica Chapman, BA, SRN, Dip N (London), RNT, is Senior Tutor (Professional Development and Post-basic Training) at Maidstone School of Nursing, and has an honorary appointment at the University of Kent at Canterbury. She was previously a tutor in the Princess Alexandra School of Nursing, The London Hospital, and later in the Staff Development Department of the Nightingale School, St Thomas' Hospital, London.

Jill Macleod Clark, BSc, PhD, SRN, is Lecturer in the Department of Nursing Studies at Chelsea College, University of London, and is currently involved in research concerned with developing methods of teaching communication skills in nursing.

Stephen Kirkham, MA, MB, BChir, MRCP, is the Medical Director of Pilgrim's Hospice, Canterbury, Kent, and has previously held both practice and research posts at St Christopher's Hospice, Sydenham, and St Joseph's Hospice, Hackney.

Daphne Hill, RMNS, SRN, RCNT, RNT, is a Nurse Tutor at the School of Nursing, St. Lawrence's Hospital, Caterham. Her ideas have contributed the basis of the discussion of the care of mentally handicapped people throughout this book and throughout the series.

Contents

Foreword to the series

This is a new series of textbooks offering a fresh approach to the study of nursing—it aims to give entrants to training, and those already qualified, an opportunity both to reflect on and to develop their own studies, and to identify their own nursing values. The text covers the material currently required by those preparing for qualification as a nurse, but it should also assist qualified nurses returning to nursing, and those wishing to gain further insight into the nursing curriculum.

The authors of each book in the series are from widely differing nursing backgrounds, and, as experienced teachers of nursing or midwifery, they are well aware of the difficulties faced by nursing students searching for meaning from a mass of factual information. The nurse has to practise in the real world, and in reality nursing students need to learn to practise with confidence and understanding. The authors have therefore collaborated to illustrate this new perspective by making full use of individual nursing care plans to present the knowledge required by the nursing student in the most appropriate and relevant way. These textbooks can therefore be used in a wide variety of nursing programmes.

Nursing training and education, and the practice of nursing—as a profession and as a career—are both affected by national and international trends. The Nurses, Midwives and Health Visitors Act 1979 in the United Kingdom, the Treaty of Rome and the European Community nursing directives 1977, as well as the deliberations and publications of the International Council of Nurses and the World Health Organization, all make an impact upon the preparation and the practice of the nurse throughout the world.

Nursing values may not have changed over the past one hundred years, but society and both the patterns of life and of care *have* changed, and are constantly changing. It is particularly important, therefore, to restate the essentials of nursing in the light of current practice and future trends.

The focus throughout this series is on nursing models of care, and on the need for continuity of care at home and in hospital. The authors place their emphasis on the *whole* person, and nursing care studies and care plans are used to promote understanding of the clinical, social, psychological and spiritual aspects of care for the individual.

Each book introduces the various aspects of the curriculum for general nursing: the special needs (1) of those requiring acute care; (2) of the elderly; (3) of children; and (4) of the mentally ill. The text on maternity and neonatal care, written by a midwifery teacher, provides the material for nursing students and would be helpful to those undertaking preparation for further health visiting education.

The authors wish to acknowledge their gratitude for the assistance they have received from members of the Editorial Board, and from all those who have contributed to their work—patients and their relatives, student and pupil nurses, qualified nurses and colleagues—too numerous to mention by name. To all those nurse teachers who have read some of the texts, offering constructive criticism and comment from their special knowledge, we offer our grateful thanks. Lastly, but by no means least, we thank Elizabeth Horne, Senior Editor of nursing books at Macmillan for her contribution to the physiology material in the text and for her perseverance and forbearance, without which the series might never have been published.

1983   Sheila Collins

Preface

An Introduction to Nursing offers the nursing student the material on which to base her future studies in order to qualify as a nurse. The characteristics of nursing, the ethical and legal aspects, and the professional responsibility of the nurse, are all explored, and the nursing student is encouraged to have a positive commitment to health and to health education, as well as a knowledge of the prevention and treatment of disease. The authors emphasise the uniqueness of each person, and the consequent need for planning the care of each patient according to his particular needs.

The text includes activities for the individual student, or for groups, in order to promote self-awareness, self-directed learning and the development of skilful communication. The reader is encouraged to relate the issues in the text to the policies, procedures and techniques used in practice and in her own nursing school. This contribution to the nursing curriculum by the nursing student forms an essential part of the text.

Nursing skills need to be learned by practice under the skilful supervision of an experienced nurse. These skills are based on a body of knowledge of nursing which needs careful study, and individual planning and effort, so that the student develops an understanding of the scientific principles underlying the art of nursing. Knowledge from many different disciplines needs interpretation in the nursing curriculum, and relationships between nursing student and teacher are important in developing this process of learning.

The nursing student, by observing the interaction between the nurse and her patient, learns to encourage each patient, so far as he is able, to contribute to the planning and evaluation of his nursing care. This text emphasises that she needs also to become actively involved in the planning, the process and the outcomes of her own nursing studies, by bringing together the knowledge she gains and the experiences she finds in the care of individual patients and their relatives.

This questioning approach to self-appraisal in practice is encouraged by references for further reading, and to research publications.

This textbook forms the central pivot for the others in the series which cover the nursing of the acutely ill, the care and welfare of the elderly, the child, the mentally ill, and maternity and neonatal care. It is the baseline—or the core—for the experience which follows, and for continuing studies throughout a nursing career.

1983

Sheila Collins
Edith Parker

Acknowledgements

The authors extend their thanks to the contributors and in particular to Daphne Hill for her help with the approach to the care of the mentally handicapped; to Anne Betts for her assistance in reading and commenting on the text; and to nursing students and colleagues for their advice and encouragement.

A note on the series style

Throughout this book, in keeping with the other titles in this series, the term *nursing student* has been used to mean *both* student or pupil nurses *and* trained nurses who are undertaking post-basic training or who are keeping up to date with the recent literature. For clarity and consistency throughout the series the nurse is described as *she*; this is done without prejudice to men who are nurses or nursing students. Similarly, the patient is sometimes referred to as *he*, when the gender is not specifically mentioned.

Care plans, which are used throughout the books in this series, are indicated by a coloured corner flash to distinguish them from the rest of the text.

Introduction

This is the introductory textbook to *The Essentials of Nursing,* and is concerned with both nursing and the nursing student. It forms an introduction to the studies which will necessarily follow if the student is to become a qualified nurse. Such studies will include the knowledge to be applied in practising the art of nursing, and those which encourage the development of personal values and attitudes which may be expressed in skilled nursing care. To deepen her understanding of the scientific basis of nursing and in planning the care of her patients, the student will be guided by her teachers in the practice of skills, and the reading and resource materials essential for self-directed learning.

Chapter 1   Nursing

Definition of Nursing

Nursing has been defined in many different words by nurses themselves, by historians, in government reports and by national and international organisations.

A well known nurse educator Virginia Henderson gave her definition in a publication for the International Council of Nurses — *Basic Principles of Nursing Care.*

'Nursing is primarily assisting the individual (sick or well) in the performance of those activities contributing to health or its recovery (or to a peaceful death) that he would perform unaided if he had the necessary strength, will or knowledge. It is likewise the unique contribution of the nurse to help the individual to be independent of such assistance as soon as possible.'

Each nurse and each nursing student has to define the meaning of the word nursing for herself, in her own words, if her course of training and her career as a nurse is to be successful.

Activity

1. Having decided to begin training to become a nurse — how do *you* define the word 'nursing'?
2. What is a nurse?
3. List the characteristics of a nurse; which do *you* consider to be important?

The core of nursing

(a) Service to others

Nursing involves service to people in preventing illness, supporting those in need and giving care to others. It involves the giving of intimate personal care at times of stress, at the edges of life and death, to the hurt, the maimed and the vulnerable. It calls for personal attributes, for the development of personal values and attitudes as well as a firm foundation of knowledge and understanding. The student of nursing requires knowledge of the scientific basis on which to make her nursing observations about her patient and on which to build her practical skills. In applying her knowledge, she learns to adapt her skills to suit the particular individual and the set of circumstances in which the care is given.

(b) Caring

Nursing as a profession, or a vocation, a career or a job of work, involves caring for people and for the individual patient as a person.

The Report of the Committee on Nursing was published in 1972, and the Chairman, Professor Asa Briggs, in that report, referred to nursing as 'the major caring profession'. There are many different forms of care; personal, social, cultural, educational, medical, legal, political, custodial, emotional and spiritual. The distinct form of care given by a nurse involves the use of her understanding and knowledge, her feeling for the person to whom the care is given and the skilful practice she uses to help a person in need. Nursing involves not only the giving of physical care, but also the giving of emotional support and understanding to her patient and his relatives or 'significant others' and the ability to encourage her patient to gain independence.

The nursing student's personal qualities and talents can be developed and deepened during the training course — few, if any, are perfect at the outset, even the 'born nurse'. Each entrant to nursing is a unique individual with differing potential. She needs to assess and recognise her own talent and attributes; and to consider for herself which aspects she needs to develop during the different stages of her course.

List in rank order, those characteristics which *you* will need to develop yourself.

(c) Human interaction

Nursing is a form of service to humanity which is essentially concerned with the interaction of human beings — the nurse or the nursing student, with her patients and their relatives, her colleagues, and all those other persons working with the patient for his benefit.

In hospital wards and departments, in the patient's home, or in a clinic or health centre, the nurse needs to listen carefully to the patient or relative and other members of the team; she needs to interpret what she hears, and to develop the art of talking to others. A nursing student needs to practise listening and replying clearly. She will often be called upon to explain treatments, or to give advice and instruction to people who are anxious or fearful. The emotional impact — fear, anxiety or insecurity — clouds the mind and understanding becomes difficult or impossible. To develop the ability to speak slowly, clearly and concisely, the nursing student needs to discover whether she can make a simple matter clear to others, and to practise until she becomes more effective in enabling others to perceive the meaning of her words.

Activity

1. Tape a conversation with a friend in which you describe something with which she is unfamiliar.
2. Play it back — listen and decide its usefulness.
3. Tape another conversation describing a course of action clearly.
4. Play it back and evaluate its strength and weakness.
5. Try again, if you still have a friend!
6. Listen to your friend describing something to you — tape this.
7. Describe to her what you have heard, taping this also.
8. Compare the two taped descriptions.

Discuss the outcome of this activity with a group of colleagues.

(d) Explanations

These are very important — patients rely on nursing staff to explain what is happening to them, and rightly expect that the nurse has the knowledge and the wish to help them.

To make the meaning clear, so that the patient can understand, it is essential to choose words that are simple, to avoid jargon and to speak clearly, repeating the words again if necessary. This is particularly important when giving information about treatment the patient is to be given, or before he goes home from the department or clinic, or before any anaesthetic is given. Research studies in nursing have shown that post-operative pain is lessened when there has been skilful nursing care and explanation about the possible effects of an operation before it has taken place (Hayward, 1975).

The tone of the voice, the time taken to speak, and the attitude or posture the nurse adopts whilst speaking to, and listening to, a patient have been shown to be important elements in the nurse–patient relationship, and in successful communication.

(e) Communicating

In word, look and touch, and by listening carefully with calm, considerate and courteous attention, communicating is an aspect of nursing which must be strongly emphasised. It is the heart of the matter — essential in caring for children and babies, for those handicapped by mental retardation, for the deaf, the elderly, for the anxious, depressed and the acutely ill, or for people with long-term illness of mind and body.

(f) Observation

Observation and accurate recording of observation form part of the nurse's care of her patient. Her sense of smell, hearing, touch, and sight will enable her to notice changes in her patient which may call for his treatment to be altered. When the patient's plan of care is being established after his admission to hospital the nurse's record of his temperature, his pulse, blood pressure, and the rate of his breathing form 'base line' observations which may be vitally important during the progress of his care. The observant nurse will note and report any change in the appearance of the patient, any change in mood, or loss of appetite, weight loss, or any unusual activity or behaviour.

Her observations — her watchfulness, will enable her to anticipate what the patient needs before he realises it.

Nursing education and training

Nursing education programmes in the UK are under statutory control, with legislation to protect the public by the provision of training for safe practice as a nurse, and to meet the UK obligations to the European Economic Community requirements.

The nursing curriculum for each school or college of nursing has to be approved and planned within guidelines which provide for both theoretical and clinical learning opportunities.

Activity

1. Read the syllabus of training for the statutory body.
2. Compare this syllabus with the outline plan of training in your own school of nursing.

The entrant to nursing training requires commitment and perseverance as well as sensitivity to the needs of others. 'Not everyone who desires to become a nurse is suitable for training' (Luckes, 1888). Physical stamina as well as health, emotional stability and an ability to get on with people are essential. Other attributes can be encouraged and developed during the training course and include gentleness, dexterity, accuracy, punctuality and confidence.

Most nursing schools and colleges require evidence of educational ability as the theoretical component of the course will be tested regularly by written and practical assessment.

(a) The learning environment

Intellectual, social and manual skills need practice for their use to be perfected. During the course of training the nursing student will have the opportunity, in a variety of different settings, with varied clinical experience, and with study sessions and visits of observation to different places, to learn to plan the use of her study time. The purpose of these placements is to deepen an awareness of the differing needs of individuals in each setting — the home, the play group, school, workplace, clinics and in hospital wards and departments. The nursing student may, therefore, learn how to modify or adapt her skills to the needs of a particular patient. She may also begin to appreciate how very complex skills are acquired and how a seemingly simple task can become difficult and intricate under certain circumstances. Each nursing student needs to accept individual responsibility for her own learning — from her experience, by asking questions, looking up references in textbooks, and by being aware that there may be more than one answer to a particular question.

(b) Nursing practice

This is grounded in theory, and nursing research projects enable the body of knowledge about nursing to grow, and to change in response to changing needs in society.

The work of nurses is often demanding, and frequently heavy. In hospital wards and departments there is often pressure of work, or the ratio of 'work to nurse power' is out of balance because of the unusual, or emergency, nature of the work. In such circumstances it is easy to assume that the nursing staff, including the nursing student, are there 'to get the work done'. The perceptive student however, will realise that within that environment lies the experience she will need to acquire in order to prepare her for her own future practice.

(c) Assessment in practice

The nurse who is qualified and in charge of a ward or department, and the teacher of nursing, will each be responsible for helping the student to progress and learn from the experience offered. It is part of the important professional responsibility of the nurse in charge to assess the potential of an individual

3

student in that particular clinical setting so that the student can concentrate her particular efforts to remedy her actions and shortcomings. Study guides and study sessions will also provide for assessment of knowledge on particular aspects of nursing, or the wider aspects of health, health education, the prevention of illness and on rehabilitation before returning to work, or on adaptations needed for the activities of daily living.

Activity

1. Make a list of the timing of the tests/assessments expected in your own school/college.
2. Add in your own school's planned programme here.
3. Devise a timetable for your own private study and written work for your tutor.

The nursing profession

'To be classified as a profession any occupation must satisfy two criteria. These are:

(i) Practical skills must be knowledge-based.
(ii) The profession must have control over the performance of its members', (Hoy and Robbins, 1979).

(a) The body of knowledge of nursing

The practice of nursing is an art — a creative activity, in which the individual nurse develops a personal approach to each person who is her patient and to each traditional task. It is also a science in that measurements of the effects of nursing can be made, trends forecast, and outcomes analysed. Research studies such as the 'Norton Scale' for the prevention of pressure sores in elderly patients in hospital (Norton *et al.*, 1975) can be used to forecast and to prevent problems which may arise under particular circumstances.

Advances in science, technology and in education assist the nursing profession to respond to, and to anticipate, changing needs within society — at local, national and international levels.

Virginia Henderson (1960), defines the unique functions of the nurse — who is:

'Temporarily the consciousness of the unconscious, the love of life for the suicidal, the leg of the amputee, the eyes of the newly blind, a means of locomotion for the infant, knowledge and confidence for the young mother, a mouthpiece for those too weak or withdrawn to speak.'

The responsibility of acquiring knowledge on which to base these various skills rests largely with the individual nurse or nursing student.

(b) Personal responsibility for professional standards

The professional responsibility of each nurse and nursing student and the standard of behaviour expected from them by those with whom they work, and those to whom they give service is a fourfold responsibility:

(i)   To the person who is the patient.
(ii) To the nurse herself.
(iii) To the colleagues with whom she works and learns.
(iv) To others in society — locally, nationally and internationally.

Such responsibility is sometimes defined in law and the legal system of the country. It is however wider than that, since it is also the standard expected of nurses by professional groups of nurses — often set down in codes of practice, or guidelines. It is therefore an ethical or moral responsibility. Ethical from the Greek ethos = character of spirit, moral from mores = the accepted standard.

This professional ethic makes demands upon the individual nurse and nursing student, which are beyond those set out in legal terms by decree or statute. For example, in free societies an individual has freedom to decide on his own actions within the law, including the right to withdraw his labour — or to strike. Nurses, like all other employees, possess that right. The integrity of the profession, the ethical code of behaviour, or practice, and the conscience of the individual nurse will dictate whether such action can be taken without harm to patients for whom and to whom that nurse is responsible.

In October 1979, the General Nursing Council for England and Wales made the following pronouncement on whether a nurse who limits or withdraws her services could face proceedings for professional misconduct.

'The Council is of the opinion that if a nurse puts the health, safety or welfare of her patients at risk by taking strike or other industrial action, she would have a case to answer on the score of professional misconduct, just as she would if the health, safety or welfare of patients were put at risk by any other action on her part.'

(c) Integrity

The nursing student needs to recognise that nursing, as a profession and an occupation, calls for integrity. A nurse is expected to hold in confidence matters related to her patient and to his personal life as well as his care and treatment; she is expected to respect the integrity of her patient. The nature of her work requires the nurse to have the ability to be true to herself, to be answerable for her own behaviour towards her patient and others, and the ability to help others to achieve the standards required, and to support their efforts to do so.

(d) Conflict

Her integrity will be taxed by conflicting demands, wishes and feelings. Nursing, which involves caring for others, brings personal rewards and satisfaction to the nurse — but it will also bring physical and emotional stress, e.g. by hard physical demands for lifting, carrying and standing, by emotional demands for the support required at moments of crisis, by the frustration of her efforts to help some patients who resist treatment or refuse to collaborate and who reject all her efforts to help. The work of the nurse may take her into situations which are often difficult, and sometimes dangerous.

The hours of work required by rotation duties, by night and day, may prevent the nursing student from enjoying the pastimes of her contemporaries.

The variety of the work, particularly during the training period, may make continual demands on the updating of knowledge and offer conflicting choices and contrasts between the demands for speed and accuracy in some acute settings, and the need for meticulous perseverance in upholding standards of care for the patients with longterm disease.

(e) Standards of care

A nurse is expected to apply her knowledge, and to practise the best possible care for her patient in the circumstances in which the care is required. In order not to be satisfied with lowered standards of care, the nurse needs to broaden her own experience by discussion with other nurses. The professional association in her own country (the Royal College of Nursing in the UK) is in contact with the national nurses' associations of other countries throughout the world by membership of the International Council of Nurses. These associations and also groups of nurses with particular specialist interests, e.g. the Geriatric Nursing Society, enable nurses to share and disseminate knowledge and to up-date each other about their practice. By this means the methods of caring, technical nursing procedures, and other aspects of nursing can be modified and adapted in response to research findings of proven worth.

Nursing calls for a deepening awareness of the importance of human relationships, an awareness of the needs of self and others and upon the ways in which human beings behave! Interpersonal skills — of contact, communication and interaction — need to be continually developed throughout the nurse's professional career.

Some aspects of the law and its relation to nursing

(a) Legal control of the profession

The right to practise as a nurse depends upon the possession of a licence granted to an individual by the registering body. In the UK, an Act of Parliament, The Nurses, Midwives and Health Visitors Act 1979, and the orders under the Act, set out the legal position by which entry to the profession is controlled. The statutory bodies — the United Kingdom Central Council, and the four National Boards for nursing, midwifery and health visiting — control the registration and conduct of members of the profession by exercising discipline, by controlling the conduct of education in nursing schools and by the carrying out of assessments and examinations.

Entry to the profession by registration, after qualification as a nurse, brings a legal as well as an ethical or moral responsibility to bear upon the nurse.

The purpose of the Act — and of the preceding Acts from 1919 onwards — is to maintain a register so that the public may know from whom safe and caring nursing service may be expected — and to protect the public by regulating the nursing profession through the disciplinary process, where necessary.

(b) The legal position of the nurse

As an individual the nurse and the nursing student is accountable for her own actions like all other members of society, in common law. As a professional nurse, qualified and responsible, or as a nursing student in training for a professional qualification, it is assumed that she has greater knowledge than the 'common man' and she is therefore expected in law to give an account of her actions based on her professional knowledge and judgement. As a person whose name appears on a register maintained on behalf of the state, she is expected to behave with due regard for the law.

(c) Professional misconduct

When a nurse pleads guilty, or is found guilty in court, of a crime against the person, she is liable to answer a charge of professional misconduct by the registering body. Such instances include for example crimes such as theft, grievous bodily harm, criminal negligence and so on, when the clerk of the court in England and Wales has to report such findings to the Registrar. A member of the public, or an employing authority may also complain about or report incidents of alleged unprofessional behaviour by qualified nurses or nursing students to the statutory bodies, leading to the investigation of possible professional misconduct. Members of the nursing profession, elected by their peers, are called upon to investigate and to examine all facets of such reports. According to the rules provided under the Act they determine whether disciplinary measures should be taken — with the possible outcome of the suspension of the nurse's licence to practise over a period of time, or the withdrawal of such licence indefinitely. Thus the professional competence of the nurse is judged by nurses — the control is in their hands.

(d) The nurse–patient relationship and the law

The law exists to protect the individual. Everyone has a right to protection from wrong-doing under the law. There are special circumstances when such rights are of great importance in nursing, either in the home or in the hospital setting, e.g. the rights of the child, of the mentally handicapped, of the mentally disturbed, of those involved in road traffic accidents and those too weak or affected by illness to protect themselves.

(e) The patient's rights

1 Consent to treatment

The patient is entitled to a full explanation of his treatment, before giving his consent for any invasion of his privacy, his possessions and his body. When the patient consults his doctor, and agrees to treatment or referral to hospital, there is an implied form of consent that he will cooperate with the medical and nursing staff and others involved in his care. If he is of age, and of sound mind, he may withdraw that implied consent if he chooses. His health and well being may be adversely affected by such action — and the doctor and nurse will have to ensure that they have clarified matters, including the possible effects on the patient. The law clearly states that it is unlawful to interfere with a person of sound mind without his consent.

2 Consent in writing

A written agreement signed by the patient is required before an operation, or before any form of investigation involving an anaesthetic, is performed. The nature and extent of the procedure should be clearly explained and written down, together with the possible effects where there is a permanent physical change in the body, e.g. the opening of the colon on to the surface of the abdomen — colostomy, or the amputation of a limb, e.g. below or above the knee; or the removal of the uterus.

3 In an emergency

When the patient's life is at stake, e.g. in railway or coach accidents, or where the patient is unconscious and the next of kin is unavailable, the surgeon may decide to operate without written consent to prevent greater danger to the patient.

4 Parental consent for minors

Parental consent is needed for treatment of a child under the age of 16. In very rare instances when this consent is withheld by parents, the child may be made a ward of court, so that the operation or treatment may be carried out. Such instances cause great concern to the individuals placed in this position, and the nursing staff have to make great efforts to prevent misunderstanding and misrepresentation. As a coordinator of the team working on behalf of the patient, the nurse plays a central role in the team's deliberations.

5 Mental Health Act

Under the provisions of the Mental Health (Amendment) Act 1982 the patient with a mental disorder has certain rights clearly written in law to protect him as an individual and to protect society from the possible effects of his disturbed behaviour whilst of unsound mind.

A patient may be admitted to a mental hospital either as a voluntary admission, or as a compulsory admission, or as an emergency compulsory admission. There are quite specific rules under the Act for patients in any of these categories. Under the Mental Health (Amendment) Act 1982 mental disorder is defined as:

    (i)   Mental illness.
    (ii) Psychopathic disorder.
    (iii) Mental impairment.
    (iv) Severe mental impairment.

Part of the Mental Health (Amendment) Act 1982 enables treatment for a patient without consent if he is admitted under section 2 — compulsory admission and detention for 28 days for assessment.

6 Patient's property

The nurse is responsible for respecting her patient and his property. In most health districts in the National Health Service in the United Kingdom there are well established policies for the care of the patient's property, i.e. his clothing and other personal possessions, jewellery, dentures, spectacles and money. In hospital wards when the patient is admitted, he is asked to hand over his property for safe keeping to the hospital authorities. A disclaimer follows usually, which indicates that this should be done in the proper manner, listed and signed, otherwise the authority will not accept responsibility in the event of loss. It is unwise for the nurse or the nursing student to undertake personal responsibility for the patient's valuables, since she is not covered by this undertaking. The 'Hospital Authorities' are those charged with safe keeping — the administrator or treasurer. A signed receipt should be given to the patient, and a copy kept in the ward to signify the articles kept for safety. When the property is returned to the patient a similar receipt should be signed for this purpose.

Activity

    1. Read the guidelines for the care of the patient's property in use in your own training school.
    2. With a colleague discuss the difficulties which may be encountered in listing his possessions.
    3. How would you describe his wallet?

4. What will you do about listing a woman's jewellery — including her wedding ring?
5. If he is admitted from a road accident and his clothing is dirty and bloodstained, what would you do?

7   The patient's will and testament

Many patients in hospital, who have never considered making a will, wish to do so for their own peace of mind, or to satisfy relatives. It is often the first time that a person has realised that it will be helpful to himself and others to indicate how he wishes to dispose of his possessions.

Making a will

A will is a legal document; it may be contested by relatives or other beneficiaries, and it is therefore very important that it is written in clear legal terms. The patient's solicitor is the best person to give professional advice. If he is not available, or if time is pressing, and if the patient is considered by the doctor to be capable of expressing his wishes clearly, the nurse may then seek the help of the health service administrator so that a simple clear statement can be drawn up for the patient. Provided that she is not mentioned in the will as a beneficiary, the nurse may act as one of the two witnesses to the signing of the will by the patient (the testator). Each of the two must witness each other's signature, and the date of the testator's signature, otherwise the will would be invalid.

It is a general rule that a nursing student should not act as a witness, and that anyone who is involved in assisting the patient should not divulge its contents. This should be done in strict confidence.

Activity

1. Read the policy regarding the making of a will in use in your training school.
2. What are the patient's rights?
3. How can the nursing student help him?
4. When a patient decides to make a will what are the responsibilities of:
   (a) the qualified nurse;
   (b) the patient's doctor;
   (c) the health service administrator?

8   Accidents or incidents

Any untoward incident occurring during the course of the nurse's work should be noted, in writing. Sometimes an incident which seems isolated, or unimportant, will assume great importance later. Nursing students, and some qualified nurses, sometimes find it difficult to express the circumstances surrounding an incident sufficiently clearly. It is necessary to indicate what occurred, when, how, who was present, and what action, if any, was taken. The reason why an incident occurred may be unknown — the fact that it happened should always be reported.

Reporting an accident

Accidents happen. Accidents affect people. The effect of the accident may be apparent — the injury may be obvious at once, or there may be no immediate apparent injury — but signs of the effect occur later.

Any accident occurring to a patient, or to a member of staff on duty, or to any visitor, should be accurately reported. Health authorities, and other employers, have agreed procedures and forms for reporting accidents. The full facts, the names of witnesses, should be indicated, and the name of the medical officer who examines the victim, together with details of any treatment required.

After an accident in hospital, or on the premises of an employing authority, has been reported, the nurse in charge, the administrator, and the doctor should examine the circumstances to see whether the cause can be found so that further such accidents may be prevented.

Activity

1. Read carefully the detailed policy for reporting an accident in use in your training school.

2. With a colleague, discuss the method of completing the form for an imaginary accident in the ward affecting:
   (a) a patient falling from a commode;
   (b) an occupational therapist falling heavily having slipped on a wet floor;
   (c) a nursing student discovering that she has given a measured medicine to the wrong patient.
3. A patient has complained that her purse containing a number of coins and notes and personal cards is missing from her locker.
   What should be the procedure following this complaint?

(f) Information which is privileged

1 Definitions

1. **Privileged** information is information held in trust, under privilege in confidence for a specific purpose.
2. A **defamatory** statement made in writing is **libel.**
3. A **defamatory** statement which is spoken is **slander.**

2 About the patient

When the patient has given the name of the person he wishes to be contacted as his next of kin, it indicates his willingness for the nurse to share information about his progress with that person. Nobody else has the right to be told about his condition or his treatment. If anyone, e.g. his employer or other enquirer wishes to have such information, the patient's permission must first be sought because this information is held in confidence under privilege. However pressing the questions, no one else can be accorded the privilege of sharing this knowledge. Sometimes members of the press seek confidential information about patients, or staff, who are celebrities. The nurse never gives such information to them, as they hold no such privilege. The administrator usually undertakes to explain this to the press and to release information only with the agreement of the patient, or his next of kin.

3 About the staff

References are often sought by prospective employers about an applicant's suitability for a post. Senior nursing staff give written replies to such requests, taking into account the assessments of the nurse, or nursing student, made by those nurses responsible for the ward or department in which the nurse has worked. Such references are written clearly, in good faith, as truthful confidential information about the person who is applying for a position of trust. Such information is also privileged.

4 Staff development

In training schools, and in most health authorities, a regular system of developing the nursing student and the trained nurse by discussion and written records is usual. These are times when each individual can be given the opportunity of discussing the work, the opportunities it offers, and of learning how to make further progress. It is the usual practice for the nursing student, and the nurse, to participate in writing such a record, and to sign the statement with her supervisor.

(g) The nurse–employer relationship and the law

1 Contracts

In the UK, registered and enrolled nurses and nursing students (i.e. student nurses and pupil nurses) are employees. In the National Health Service they are the employees of the local health authority (called an Area (AHA) in Scotland, a district (DHA) in England, and a Health Board in Northern Ireland).

Under the law each employee is entitled to a contract, setting out the terms of employment — what the employee can expect from her employer, and vice versa. The details to be covered in the contract, in writing, include:

(a) the date of commencement, the place of employment;
(b) the grade of employment, details of pay scale;
(c) the holiday entitlement, and the superannuation regulations;
(d) the grievance procedure and how it works.

Most contract forms draw the attention of the employee to the place where copies of the full details of the terms and conditions of service agreed by the Nurses and Midwives Whitley Council can be found, since not every aspect can be enumerated on the contract form.

2 The nursing student – employee contract

In addition to the above details, the contract for a nursing student should also include the following:

(a) the specified length of training, since it is for a fixed term;
(b) the regulations for training imposed by the statutory body controlling professional training;
(c) the assessments and examinations to be passed during the course.

The statutory body requires evidence of the progress of the nursing student towards the satisfactory completion of the training period. The policy of the training school to meet these requirements — regarding entry, number of attempts and the procedure in the event of failure to pass these assessments and examinations — should be available with the contract, and an outline curriculum or plan of training.

3 The employer's rights in the contract

The employer has a right to expect the employee to behave competently and to be trustworthy. If an employer is dissatisfied with the work of an employee, he can warn that there is cause for concern, recommend further effort, and set a time limit for improvement. Such warnings may be given formally — verbally or in writing in the presence of a representative of a trade union, or a friend — at the choice of the employee.

Most health authorities list actions which would be taken as examples of breach of contract warranting summary dismissal, e.g. deliberate action against a patient, misuse of drugs, intoxication on duty, assault to others on the premises and so on.

4 The nursing student and the grievance procedure

The guidelines for invoking the grievance procedure will be laid down by the employing authority — together with an agreed method of dealing with the grievance stage by stage.

As an employee the nursing student who feels aggrieved has the right to discuss this, and gain the help of the accredited representative of her trade union. As a student in training under the regulations of the statutory body and of the training school, she may also discuss her problems with one of her teachers, or a registered nurse, to clarify the local policy, if she so wishes.

During her clinical experience, the nursing student is accountable to her ward/department sister or charge nurse, for the participation in the care of patients. A misdemeanour on duty during her work may therefore be the reason for counselling or for a reprimand, or by a report to the nursing officer. Failure to make progress with studies, or a misdemeanour occurring during study sessions, may be the reason for counselling or for a reprimand by her teacher of nursing. A verbal or formal written warning, setting the timescale for improvement, may follow either of these events. A nursing student who considers that there is reason to invoke the grievance procedure to challenge such decisions, has the right of appeal to the head of the training school.

5 Abortion Act 1967

Section 4(i) of the Abortion Act states:

'No person shall be under any duty, whether by contract or by any statutory or other legal requirement to participate in any treatment authorised by this act to which there is conscientious objection. Providing that in any legal proceedings the burden of proof of conscientious objection shall rest on the person claiming it.'

It is, therefore, advisable that any nurse or nursing student, with strongly held beliefs which make her unwilling to participate in such treatment, should write formally, at the outset of her employment, to her employer asking for this to be recorded and respected.

Nursing students will recognise the dilemma which exists between personal and professional ethics and religious conviction on such an issue. The conservation of life is one of the ethical principles of nursing, yet so is the relief of suffering, and the nurse has to be sensitive to social needs, and the pressures upon the individual. Although the legal position of the nurse and student is clear from the above statement, the personal pressures upon those who opt out from such treatments, leaving others to undertake such work, can be considerable. When the life of a patient is in danger, however, there is no doubt that the nurse cannot leave her patient without alternative support and care whatever her own personal beliefs.

It may be helpful to consider here that this is the only legal ruling regarding the protection of those who choose not to take part in nursing treatment. There is no such protection for nurses, or nursing students, who dislike certain aspects of their work, e.g. a certain type of ward or department, a particular type of procedure, or a particular class of patient and so on. If this presents a problem, the nursing student should discuss it with the nurse in charge, or with her teacher of nursing. A qualified nurse may be wise to seek alternative employment if she finds the work distasteful.

6 The Health and Safety at Work Act 1974

Under this act, both employees and employers have a duty to ensure that the health, welfare and safety of employees is safeguarded. This places on employers the duty to set down the policy, and the guidelines, for practice of any procedures which may affect the health and safety of those at work. It also places on those who work with equipment, or in hazardous situations, the duty of carrying out the agreed procedures correctly. Any employee failing to take proper care within the guidelines may be called to account by his employer.

Activity

1. Read the policy guidelines in your own training school for isolation of an infectious patient.
2. Consider your responsibilities for protecting yourself and others from this infectious disease.
3. How will you explain to the domestic assistant cleaning the room and to the family and friends visiting the patient, what is required from them?

7 Trade Union and Labour Relations Act 1974

Every employee has the right not to be unfairly dismissed, and this act sets out her right of appeal against a dismissal thought to be unfair. An appeal will be heard by an impartial tribunal.

8 Employment Protection Act 1975

This act protects the rights of employees who are members of trades unions. It covers the right of an employee to participate in such activities, for accredited representatives to have time allowed in preparation for such duties and to be consulted and participate in staff/management discussions.

All these aspects of law are important for nursing staff in their work, and for nursing students undergoing training. There are many others — particularly those relating to the individual client or patient — with which she will need to become familiar throughout her career. The professional conduct of the nurse and her preparation and education, are under the control of the statutory body responsible for issuing her licence to practise as a nurse.

References

Briggs, A., Report of the Committee on Nursing, Cmnd 5115, HMSO, 1972
Hayward, J., *Information — A Prescription against Pain,* The Study of Nursing Care, Project Reports, Series 1, RCN, 1975
Henderson, V., *Basic Principles of Nursing Care,* ICN, 1960
Hoy, R. and Robbins, J., *The Profession of Nursing,* McGraw-Hill, 1979
Luckes, E., *General Nursing,* Kegan Paul, 1888
Norton, D., McClaren, R. and Exton-Smith, A.N., *An Investigation of Geriatric Nursing Problems in Hospital,* Churchill Livingstone, 1975

Further reading

Hector, W., *The Work of Mrs Bedford Fenwick and the Rise of Professional Nursing,* RCN, 1970

McFarlane, J., *The Proper Study of the Nurse,* RCN, 1970

Quinn, S. (Ed.), *Nursing in the European Community,* Croom Helm, 1980

Report of the Committee on Nursing, Cmnd 5115, HMSO, 1972

Wakefield, R., *The Law and the Nurse,* Hodder and Stoughton, 1974

Whincup, M.H., *Legal Rights and Duties in the Medical and Nursing Service,* Vol. 5, Ravenswood, 1975

Chapter 2   Health

Introduction

The International Council of Nurses' meeting in Mexico in 1973 adopted the following code of ethical concepts applied to nursing.

'The fourfold responsibility of the nurse is
- to promote health;
- to prevent illness;
- to restore health;
- to alleviate suffering.'

Health has been defined by the World Health Organization (1947) as 'A state of complete physical, mental and social well being, not merely the absence of disease or infirmity'.

This definition is widely used in nursing schools and merits careful thought.

Activity

1. Are there any additional aspects that you think are important in the definition?
2. How would you define 'disease'?
3. What is 'infirmity'?

An alternative definition has been given by Kathleen Mansfield: 'By health, I mean the power to live a full adult living breathing life in close contact with what I love. I want to be all that I am capable of becoming'.

Each person is responsible for his own life, health and safety — provided that he has the capacity for reasoned behaviour. Choices between two or more courses of action have to be made, and decisions taken daily which affect the person's lifestyle and his behaviour. The role of the nurse is to enable the person to perceive the possible outcomes of each decision.

The promotion of health

The basic physical needs for health in the human being are sometimes likened to those of other members of the animal kingdom: air, water, food, shelter and warmth, rest and sleep, activity and sexual expression. To these — for the person — should be added social and emotional needs, the need for love and

Death of a spouse	Retirement
Divorce	Illness of close family member, or close friend
Marital separation/Marital problems	Sexual difficulties
Death of close friend, or close family member	Change in financial state
Personal injury or illness	Change in working conditions/hours of work/place of work
Marriage	Change in responsibilities at work
Loss of work/occupation/job	Change in living conditions/place of residence
Redundancy	

Figure 2.1   Events which may lead to stress in the life span of an individual

approval, for intellectual or spiritual refreshment, and creativity, for personal satisfaction, self-esteem and achievement, or self-actualisation. Many theories exist about these human needs and the relationship between the physiological needs for survival and the continuation of the species and the psychological or emotional needs of the individuals and groups. These aspects of social, psychological and physiological needs will be further developed throughout the course of nursing.

Activity

1. List other situations which *you* find stressful.
2. Compare and discuss the list with your colleagues.

Disability and health

A person who has a disability is still a member of the society in which he lives, and he has the same needs for healthy living as everyone else. He is healthy, or unhealthy. Such individuals need to be independent — to do as much as possible for themselves. Support from family, friends and neighbours, and from nurses, should enable the person to be independent and to live within the limits of his disability.

(a) Physical disability

Some people are born with a physical defect — abnormalities of the limbs, eyes, or skin ('port wine stains'), or other congenital abnormalities.

Some people become crippled or disabled by accidents, or by disease in later life.

In 1981, the International Year of the Disabled, attention was focused on the needs of these people, particularly on their need for a 'normal' healthy environment, for satisfying personal, social and sexual relationships and for mobility. When a physically handicapped person is ill, the nurse should be particularly careful to arrange for him to have personal freedom, mobility and independence, and to avoid over-protection, or patronising assumptions that he is unable to look after himself.

Activity

1. Consider the difference between the use of the terms:
   (a) 'The disabled'.
   (b) 'Person with a disability'.
2. List the physical achievements of people with disability that you have read about in books or newspapers.
3. What arrangements are there to encourage greater independence of a person without legs in your own locality?
4. What social benefits are available for people with physical disability?

(b) Mental handicap

A person who has a mental handicap is someone who has not the mental capacity which is accepted as normal in their own society. The term is a convenient social and administrative one covering a large number of conditions which affect the person's ability to learn and to reason. It is not an illness which can be treated and cured.

Mental impairment is a relatively new term used in the Mental Health (Amendment) Act 1982 and covers the words 'mental deficiency' formerly used in Scotland, 'mental subnormality' in England and Wales, and 'mental retardation' in other countries. It is usually defined by measuring the intelligence quotient (IQ). The average IQ is taken to be 100; anyone with an IQ of 50–70 is said to have a mild degree of mental impairment, and anyone with an IQ below 50 is considered to be severely mentally impaired.

1 Causes of mental handicap

Most of the conditions which lead to mental handicap are determined before birth, or in the early weeks of life. Faulty development during pregnancy may cause physical as well as mental disability or handicap.

Mentally handicapped people will never be cured, but measures to prevent handicap are beginning to become clearer, and in the last ten years there have been developments in understanding the needs of the mentally handicapped for proper training and education to cope with the ordinary skills of everyday living which most people take for granted.

Mildly mentally handicapped people may fit so neatly into their own society that nobody realises that they are anything except 'a bit slow'.

The Warnock Report (1978) recommended that mildly and moderately mentally handicapped children should, wherever possible, be taught in ordinary schools, mixing with 'normal' children, to encourage their development, and that there should be no segregation for these mentally handicapped children in special schools.

ESN schools are special schools for slow learners and there are 51 000 places in such schools in England and Wales, and a further 11 000 on waiting lists.

An exact cause of mental handicap is often difficult to find. There are nearly 300 known causes, but in only 35% of known instances of handicap, can an exact cause be found. It is seldom true that mental handicap is inherited from handicapped parents, which was previously thought to be so. Inherited inborn errors in genetic makeup, faulty development during pregnancy, difficulties during childbirth, and social factors, as well as the effects of disease are all included in the large variety of causes.

Social factors

Prematurity, and malnutrition in infancy can retard mental development. Babies who weigh less than the average at birth tend to be below average at normal milestones of development. Overcrowding, or poor housing conditions, may mean that there is little individual attention for the baby. Studies have shown that children born in impoverished or specially deprived homes have less chance to develop their potential. When the mother goes out to work alternative child minders may fail to encourage the individual child. If they then go to overcrowded or inadequately staffed schools they may then continue to lose ground.

Disease

1. Disease of the pregnant woman may cause mental handicap. Rubella, or german measles is one example. There is a one in ten chance of a handicap in the child if the mother develops this disease in the early months of pregnancy. There is now a vaccine offered to all teenage girls to prevent the likelihood of this occurring. The pregnant woman can choose to have an abortion if she has rubella during early pregnancy.
2. Disease of the child may cause mental handicap, e.g. inflammation of the coverings of the brain — meningitis, or of the brain itself — encephalitis, may also cause handicap as a complication of the disease. It is a possible complication of measles — for which immunisation is now available.

Brain damage

This may occur during development, or at birth or in the first few weeks of life. Not *all* babies injured before or during birth suffer from mental handicap: it has been estimated that approximately half those with cerebral palsy — spastics — are mentally handicapped, a quarter of whom are severely mentally handicapped, as well as having physical handicap.

Hydrocephalus, or 'water on the brain' may be a cause — unless treatment is undertaken early to release the blockage caused to the flow of cerebrospinal fluid, and so to prevent the back pressure exerted by the fluid on the brain substance.

Chromosome abnormalities

It is now possible to detect abnormality in the chromosomes before the child is born. In every 700 births there is likely to be one abnormality known as Down's syndrome (Mongolism). The likelihood of this incidence increases with the age of the mother from 1 in 2400 births if the mother is 20, to 1 in 100 if the mother is aged 40.

Errors of metabolism

There are errors in the metabolism of some infants, which interfere with normal growth and development. One example is phenylketonuria, a disease where an infant cannot cope with an ordinary diet; a diet low in phenylalanine may prevent such babies from developing severe mental handicap. Another example, fortunately rare, is caused by failure of development of the thyroid gland, leading to failure of growth. If the baby is treated with thyroxine, and if this is taken continually, metabolism may be corrected, and mental handicap may be prevented.

2 Summary

Mental handicap is not itself a disease, and the problems produced by handicap are personal, social and educational.

In 1978 the Report of the Committee of Enquiry into Mental Handicap and Nursing Care under the chairmanship of Mrs Peggy Jay was published. This far-reaching report, suggesting fundamental changes in the approach to mental handicap, and in the provision of care for these individuals, was the subject of much debate by the nursing and medical professions, by social workers and teachers, and by all those keenly interested in society's obligations to those needing special care and consideration. Controversy continues regarding some of the recommendations in this report, but there is undoubtedly a need for continuing discussion by all those people concerned with mentally handicapped children and adults.

Observation, patience and tolerance are especially important when a mentally handicapped person is admitted to an acute ward for surgical treatment or for investigation of a medical problem. Chronological age is no guide to the 'age' of the person in terms of behaviour to be expected. The nurse's kindness and good humour are appreciated, and the non-verbal cues which the nurse gives are very important for such patients to feel a real sense of security in a new and bewildering environment.

Medical and nursing care may be helpful, not only in preventing or treating physical outcomes of handicap, but also in providing support and care to relieve pressures on the parents, and to prevent family and social breakdown, at times of stress. The stress caused to parents in caring for a mentally handicapped child may affect the marriage, and the siblings. But it is often even more distressing for ageing parents who wonder who will care for an older mentally handicapped son or daughter, when they can no longer do so. The development of small sheltered homes within the locality for such persons owes much to pressure groups in the United Kingdom.

Further reading

Report of the Committee of Enquiry into Mental Handicap and Nursing Care, Cmmd. 7468 (2 vols), HMSO, 1978

Health provision

The World Health Organization has drawn attention to the fact that there is a direct relationship between the health of a population and a pure water supply, sanitation, shelter, and food of the right type and quantity. In western countries the provision of resources to meet the needs of society is determined by political action, supported by governmental agencies and the law. The provision of a water supply, of clean food, adequate drainage and the treatment of sewage, the prevention of air pollution, and of financial assistance for those in need, for the old and those who are frail, or disabled, is undertaken by the State, with monies provided from the public purse — by revenue and taxation. In 1877 Disraeli said 'The health of the people is really the foundation upon which all their happiness and all their power as a state depend'.

Social, cultural, religious and ethnic differences should always be respected by a nurse — particularly when promoting health, or giving advice on the prevention of disease and when nursing the patient.

1. Consider the differences in housing between the district where your school is sited, and a rural area where you have spent a holiday.
2. What effect does this have on the health of a family?

Measurement of health

The measurement of health in a country, or local community depends upon the data available. In the UK information is recorded by the Registrar General, and consists of vital statistics.

Registration of birth, notification of birth, registration of still birth, of death and the notification of certain communicable diseases are legal requirements. The population census includes details of each member of the household, e.g. name, age, sex, occupation, qualifications, means of transport to work, the type of household accommodation, number of rooms, bathroom/shower, cooker and so on. From the census figures, the Registrar General classifies the population into different social classes, based upon the occupation of the chief wage earner in the family. This enables comparisons to be made regarding the incidence of disease, or the cause of death between differing groups in society.

Classification according to occupation

Non-Manual: Class I. Professional occupations, e.g. lawyers and doctors.
                    Class II. Managerial and other occupations, e.g. nurses and teachers.
                    Class III.N Skilled non-manual occupations, e.g. clerks, shop assistants.

Manual: Class III.M Skilled manual occupations, coal face workers.
              Class IV. Partly skilled manual occupations, e.g. bus conductors.
              Class V. Unskilled occupations, e.g. railway porters.

Population trends and social trends can be used to assess needs, and in planning for the future use of resources.

Health education

Health education begins in the family, where social customs and habits are developed during the process of early socialisation. Differing standards are set according to the social group which determines such acceptable 'norms' according to the mores of that society. Nurseries, schools and colleges continue the development of positive or negative attitudes to health. The media, advertising, and social pressures provide conflicting information on aspects of health and healthy living. The nurse is often called upon to identify the priorities for her colleagues, and for those whom she meets in social context, and she is expected to advise her patient and his relatives on the promotion or restoration of his health.

Activity

What aspects of health do you consider need emphasis:
(a) To young schoolchildren?   (c) To pregnant women?
(b) To adolescents?   (d) To an elderly widower living alone?

Occupational health

Health education and the promotion of health may be continued at work. Many commercial firms, industrial concerns and some health authorities provide an occupational health service for their employees. In such a service the occupational health nurse plays an important part in helping individuals to promote their own health and to prevent illness and disability due to the nature of their work.

Further reading

Advisory Committee on Alcoholism, Report on Prevention, DHSS, 1977
Anderson Digby, C. (Ed.), *Health Education in Practice,* Croom Helm, 1979
Carnana, S. and Buttimore, A., *Nurses' Handbook on Alcohol and Alcoholism,* Medical Council on Alcoholism and Queen's Institute for District Nursing, 1974
Sutherland, I. (Ed.), *Health Education, Perspectives and Choices,* Allen and Unwin, 1977

Legislation and health

To protect the public there are acts of Parliament and statutory instruments concerned with health in the UK, e.g. the Health and Safety at Work Act 1974 sets out to identify the responsibilities of both employers and employees for the promotion of safe practices at work to promote health. Environmental health in a locality is the responsibility of environmental health officers working for a local authority; they ensure that the provision of a series of acts to protect the public are being applied, e.g. the Clean Air Act 1956, 1961 and 1974 and the Food and Drugs Act 1968–1973.

The National Health Service Act 1948 is concerned with the promotion of health and the prevention of disease, as well as with the provision of services for those who are ill — either with acute or long-term illness, or who need rehabilitation to return to work, or to their former lifestyle. Services provided under the National Health Service are the responsibility of health authorities — in Scotland, Wales and Northern Ireland such authorities cover different areas of the country, whilst in England there are 14 regional health authorities, each with a varying number of district authorities to administer the provisions of the act for the locality.

All the health authorities are charged with the provision of:

1. Antenatal care, midwifery and postnatal services to promote health for mother and baby, by midwives and health visitors.
2. Health screening and health teaching by school nurses and by health visitors for children of pre-school age, for families or for vulnerable groups in society, e.g. the frail elderly, tuberculosis contacts.
3. Home nursing services by nurses trained in home nursing (district nurses) for those who are ill at home, with the teaching of relatives and support staff regarding the prevention of further disability.
4. Family planning services, provided in midwifery units, in health clinics, by nurses, midwives or health visitors, and by general practitioners in their surgeries or health centres.
5. The provision of nursing advice to all nursing homes within the locality of the health authority, i.e. those run by the health authority, and those residential homes run by the Social Services Department of the local authority. The registration of private nursing homes within the boundaries of the authority is vested in the health authority when the standard of nursing care, staffing levels and equipment, are taken into account, and advice on nursing matters is therefore very important.

The emphasis on the promotion of health, the prevention of illness and on primary health care was the subject of government reports and publications and is promoted by the World Health Organization ('Prevention and Health: Everybody's Business, 1976').

Further reading

DHSS, *Prevention and Health: Everybody's Business,* HMSO, 1976

The nursing student and the promotion of health

In matters of health, the individual person has to make choices between healthy and harmful practices. The purpose of teaching is to ensure that the facts, the pros and cons of a particular behaviour are understood, so that the person can make a reasoned choice. The student has to learn to play the role of health educator. It is the nurse's responsibility as a health teacher to make sure that the patient has the full facts and knowledge relevant to the situation, and that he perceives the effect of his decision on his lifestyle and practices, which not only affect himself but others as well.

The public image of a nurse is someone who helps to care for and cure the sick in hospital, not someone who helps in the prevention of ill health by promoting healthy practices, who helps patients and clients make their own reasoned decisions about their own lifestyles.

The candidate entering nursing often has this idea of the wider role of the nurse, and therefore she has to learn to become a health teacher. In accepting this role, she will realise that she has to adapt or modify her own practices to become a role model for the patients/clients in her charge. For example, the patient will not take much note of the nurse who is suggesting that he should give up smoking because of the adverse effects on his lungs, if she talks to him with smoke-laden breath. Likewise, a patient may feel unhappy about accepting advice on the need for a reducing diet from a perspiring, obviously overweight nurse. The nurse, as an individual, must of course make her own decisions about her *own* lifestyle, while remembering that she has a professional role with its responsibilities.

(a) Teaching about health

If she decides, for example, to continue smoking, the student must appreciate that she must be prepared to be challenged by the patient, and to be able to discuss with him the reasons for her behaviour.

The nursing student should also learn about how to prevent disease spreading, and to promote health under adverse conditions. Legislation cannot ensure the prevention of illness, nor outbreaks of disease in times of natural disaster — earthquakes, floods, eruptions of volcanoes, in times of drought, famine, bush fires and wars. At such times the nurse needs to apply her knowledge about preventing contamination of water supplies by sewage, preventing food from contamination by flies, insects and animals and by burning refuse.

The nurse who teaches the young mother to boil water to make it safe for use in feeding a sick child, who teaches others the value of fresh air and ventilation, as a stimulus for activity in homes, schools and hospital wards is also acting as a health teacher.

Outbreaks of disease may occur wherever large numbers of people are gathered together in limited space, with limited facilities, and where food preparation and service, and sanitation arrangements, are stretched to the limit; for example, at festivals, marches, camping grounds and pleasure boats.

The speed of travel, and the size of aircraft, has increased the possible spread of virulent disease from one part of the world to another by people who are 'carriers' — either incubating or suffering from a disease or infection — in close proximity to others.

Air conditioning plant and showers or swimming baths, which bring progress and comfort to modern living, may also present hazards to health by disseminating water-borne disease, e.g. Legionnaire's Disease.

Health and the human body

The nursing student needs an accurate knowledge of the way that the health of the human body is maintained. She will need this knowledge to keep herself healthy, to teach patients and others about health and prevention of disease and disability, and in her care of the patient and his relatives.

Scientific advances are continually revealing to us more about the way the body works; reading and studying up-to-date material is therefore essential throughout a nursing career. During the training course the student needs to deepen her knowledge of each of the systems of the body, the interaction between them and the interaction between mind and body. Only thus will she be able to understand the needs of her patient, the *symptoms* (see p. 20) caused by illness, and the effects of disease upon the patient, his relatives or the society in which he lives. Such knowledge is essential when assessing needs before formulating a plan for the nursing care of any patient.

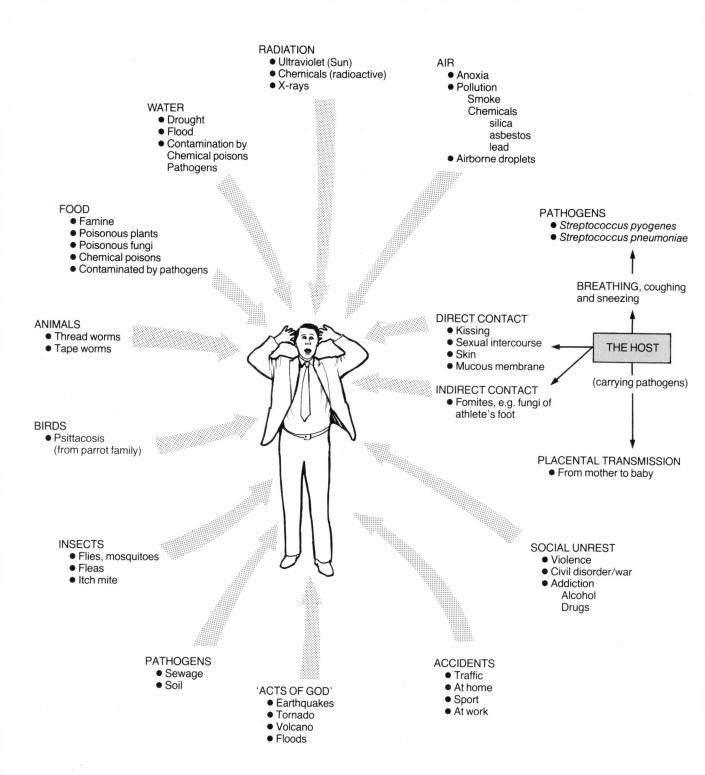

RADIATION
- Ultraviolet (Sun)
- Chemicals (radioactive)
- X-rays

AIR
- Anoxia
- Pollution
  Smoke
  Chemicals
    silica
    asbestos
    lead
- Airborne droplets

WATER
- Drought
- Flood
- Contamination by
  Chemical poisons
  Pathogens

PATHOGENS
- *Streptococcus pyogenes*
- *Streptococcus pneumoniae*

FOOD
- Famine
- Poisonous plants
- Poisonous fungi
- Chemical poisons
- Contaminated by pathogens

BREATHING, coughing
and sneezing

ANIMALS
- Thread worms
- Tape worms

DIRECT CONTACT
- Kissing
- Sexual intercourse
- Skin
- Mucous membrane

THE HOST

INDIRECT CONTACT
- Fomites, e.g. fungi of
  athlete's foot

(carrying pathogens)

BIRDS
- Psittacosis
  (from parrot family)

PLACENTAL TRANSMISSION
- From mother to baby

INSECTS
- Flies, mosquitoes
- Fleas
- Itch mite

SOCIAL UNREST
- Violence
- Civil disorder/war
- Addiction
  Alcohol
  Drugs

PATHOGENS
- Sewage
- Soil

'ACTS OF GOD'
- Earthquakes
- Tornado
- Volcano
- Floods

ACCIDENTS
- Traffic
- At home
- Sport
- At work

Figure 2.2   *The hazards to the individual from his environment*

Activity

Consider the other environmental conditions which would endanger the health
of the individual. When you have had time to consider this, see p. 27.

Definition

Symptoms: These are characteristic of a particular disease or condition about
  which a patient may complain, because he feels them or feels the limitations
  to his daily life that they cause.
For example, he may complain of a sore throat, or a cough, of pain on moving
  a joint, of discomfort after meals, or nausea and so on, of tiredness, lassitude
  or weakness.

The observant nurse may also notice certain aspects of a particular patient's
appearance, behaviour or changes in his bodily functions.

These are called signs, and the doctor examining a patient looks for certain signs which enable him to diagnose the illness or condition, e.g. pallor, rashes, changes in the composition of the urine.

The body as a whole

At this introductory stage of training it is the way in which the body works as a whole in health that is important. It needs careful study to appreciate how the activities are kept in balance — no part working in isolation, the action of one part affecting others. For convenience, textbooks about anatomy and physiology sometimes divide the body into systems for description — but the nursing student needs to approach her own studies remembering that each system is only part of a whole and that all bodily systems are interdependent.

Definition

Anatomy: The study of the structure of the healthy human body.
Physiology: The study of the functions of the healthy human body.
Pathology: The study of disease processes.
Physiopathology: The study of disease processes affecting the functions of the human body.

Sometimes a mechanistic model is used and the human body is likened to a machine, or a factory, which uses raw materials and energy to maintain and renew itself and to make products resulting in by-products and waste materials for disposal. One of the most active organs in such activity is the liver, which is a vital organ, essential for life and health.

Definition

System: A system of the body has special functions and is made up of several organs, e.g. the skeletal system.
Organ: An organ of the body is made up of different types of tissue to perform a special, vital function in the body. The organs of the digestive system are: the gastro-intestinal tract (mouth, oesophagus, the stomach, duodenum), the liver, gall-bladder and its ducts, the pancreas, small intestine, large intestine, rectum and anus.

The living cell

(a) Cells

The smallest unit of the body is the cell, a collection of protoplasm — living matter which contains a nucleus. The shape and appearance of cells vary according to the work they are called upon to do. A collection of similar cells with the same function is called a tissue.

The cells of the living body are constantly active to maintain their protoplasm in a state of 'dynamic equilibrium'.

(b) Fluid: cellular and tissue fluid

For all this activity, the cells need water. Without water the cells and the human body will die. The tissue fluid in the spaces between the cells is the medium in which the chemical changes take place, i.e. for the cell to receive the nutrients in solution which it needs, for the cell to select materials with which to make products and to renew its protoplasm, or to reproduce. The tissue fluid receives from the cell its products and waste materials, to be taken away.

Tissue fluid contains oxygen and nutrients — water, mineral salts, vitamins, glucose, amino acids and fatty acids. It also contains enzymes and hormones which act as chemical catalysts enabling chemical changes to occur in their presence, while remaining unchanged. Oxidation of glucose in the presence of insulin releases energy for the cell's activities. Carbon dioxide and water are produced during oxidation and these, with other unwanted materials and waste materials or products from the cells are transferred from the tissue fluid to the circulatory system. In the circulatory system those materials are carried to all other parts of the body, either for use, or to be converted to other materials in the liver, or eliminated from the body by the kidneys, the skin, the lungs or the intestinal tract.

1. *Protoplasm:* A living substance of which the cell is made, soft, colourless, jelly-like. Contains:
● Water, and organic and inorganic salts
● Lipids (fatty substances)
● Amino acids (nitrogenous substances from protein)
● Compounds
Cytoplasm: the protoplasm of the cell body
Nucleoplasm: The protoplasm of the nucleus of the cell

2. *Cell membrane:* A fine membrane -
● Protein and lipids with tiny holes, allowing diffusion to occur from a higher to a lower concentration
● Lipids allow other substances to be dissolved and carried across the membrane
● A carrier system within the membrane allows other substances to be picked up across the membrane

3. Chromatin: Threads within the nucleoplasm carry the genes, made up of DNA (deoxyribonucleic acid). These genes are linked together to form pairs of chromosomes — 46 in each cell as 23 pairs

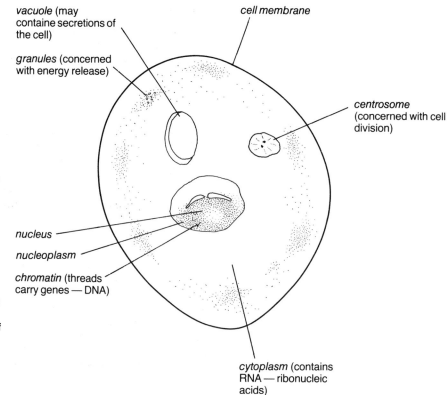

Figure 2.3 A simple cell

It is essential for life and health to be maintained that a balance should be achieved between the amount of fluid taken into the body plus the amount gained during the activities within the cells, and the amount of fluid eliminated from the body. The kidneys play a vital role in regulating the amount of fluid eliminated or retained in order to keep the composition of the circulating blood constant in health.

(c) Controlling the activities of the cells

A complex mechanism controls the functions of all the cells in the tissues of each system of the body. The objective is to keep the internal environment of the body in a state of equilibrium and in balance with the external environment. The term used to describe this is homeostasis. To achieve this there is a feedback system for the exchange of information, with checks and balances, so that messages are constantly being relayed to and from the different parts of the body to maintain this balance. Two systems of the body work closely together to exercise this control — the nervous system and the endocrine system (the ductless glands which produce chemical messengers called hormones). Hormones are carried in the bloodstream to the tissues where they influence the chemical changes carried out within the cells. For example insulin, a hormone produced by the special cells in the pancreas is carried in the blood to the body cells so that energy may be obtained for cell activity during oxidation. When there is an increasing need for energy by oxidation the level of insulin in the blood rises to enable glucose and fatty acids to be utilised, and for the release of glucose from the liver where it is stored as glycogen.

1 Metabolism

Metabolism is a term used to describe all the chemical changes taking place within the body.

Anabolism

Anabolism is the term used to describe cell activities which result in the building up of substances into protoplasm or to renew cells, or to make hormones, or other useful products such as sebum from the sebaceous glands in the skin, or digestive juices in the gastrointestinal tract, or mucus from the mucous membrane in the mouth.

Catabolism

Catabolism is a term used for all the activities in which breakdown occurs, e.g. when the cell protoplasm is broken into its component parts or when it is making waste products, and the chemical changes occurring when the glucose and fatty acids are oxidised to provide energy and from which carbon dioxide and water results.

The rate at which metabolism occurs will vary from one individual to another, it will also vary according to the amount of energy required by the body, and according to the amount of activity within the cells. The hormone thyroxine from the thyroid gland plays a part in the controlling mechanism for the basal rate of metabolism. The **basal metabolic rate** (BMR) is at its lowest with the body at rest lying flat in the early morning following a night's rest, and without food for 12 hours.

(d) Diffusion

Diffusion is the term used to describe the physical process by which dissolved substances move from a higher to a lower concentration to achieve equilibrium in the solution.

This is not a rapid process, as you can illustrate by dropping a little coloured ink into a glass of water.

Some of the dissolved nutrients inside the gut pass by diffusion into the tissue fluid, lymph, and blood vessels into the circulation. The increased surface area of the lining of the intestines increases the opportunity for this to occur.

Oxygen and respiration

(a) Oxygen

Oxygen is essential for human life as most of the activities within the cells require oxygen to oxidise glucose for energy, which results in the production of carbon dioxide and water. Without oxygen the body dies, therefore breathing is a vital function and maintaining a clear airway is an essential first aid measure. The air which is breathed into the lungs (inspired) contains approximately 21% oxygen. The oxygen in the air sacs (the alveoli) of the lungs passes in solution into the blood in the capillaries — which surround the alveoli — by the process of diffusion. Carbon dioxide from the blood capillaries diffuses through into the alveoli in solution, to be breathed out together with water. The large surface area of the alveoli in the lungs enables this exchange of gases to occur more easily.

(b) Breathing

Breathing is a muscular activity, involving the diaphragm, a large muscle separating the chest and abdominal cavities, and the muscles between the ribs. Chemical stimulation of the autonomic nervous system enables the respiratory centre in the brain to maintain respiration. The rising level of carbon dioxide carried in the blood triggers messages which stimulate the centre, altering the rate and depth of respiration. Breathing is, therefore, only partially under the control of the individual's will by the central nervous system — as those who learn to sing or swim soon have to learn.

Nutrition

This may be described as the sum of the processes by which a living organism receives materials from its environment and uses them for its own activities.

Food is vital for living organisms, but although the human body cannot live without water it can live for some time without food. Health requires a balanced diet. Each person requires to achieve a balance between the amount of food eaten and the amount of energy required for work or any activity to be undertaken.

The type of food, as well as the correct amount, is important for health, and for healthy growth and reproduction. The diet therefore must contain the essential food factors. Dietetics is the application of the science of nutrition to the selection and preparation of food in the construction of diets.

Activity

List the types of food you have eaten during the past 24 hours.
1. What was the calorific value of the food you have eaten?
2. Look up the average amount of calories (or joules) required by an active adult of your own age.
3. What proportion of fat, protein and carbohydrate did you eat at each meal?
4. Which vitamins did your diet contain — what is the function of each?
5. What was the amount of your fluid intake?

(a) Digestion

The process of taking food (ingestion), chewing (mastication) and swallowing begins a series of chemical changes and muscular action in the walls of the gastrointestinal tract. This muscular movement is called peristalsis and the action mixes the chewed food material with digestive juices from the glands in the mouth, the stomach and small intestine, and with mucus secreted by the glands in the mucous membrane in the tract. In addition, bile produced in the liver, and stored in the gall bladder is carried down the common bile duct into the upper part of the small intestine – the duodenum. Bile contains chemicals which emulsify fats making it easier for digestive enzymes to break them down into fatty acids and glycerol. Bile also colours the contents of the tract giving the normal brown colour to faeces. Digestive enzymes from the pancreas are also carried down the pancreatic duct direct to the duodenum (not to be confused with the hormones secreted by the Islets of Langerhans in the pancreas directly into the circulatory system, namely insulin and glucagon).

Digestion results from chemical changes occurring in the tract in the presence of digestive enzymes. These chemicals render the food into small components called nutrients: starches and sugars (carbohydrates) become glucose; fats become fatty acids and glycerol; meat, fish, eggs, milk, pulses (proteins) become amino acids. These nutrients, together with vitamins and mineral salts and water, are then ready for absorption in solution.

Activity

List the digestive enzymes responsible for converting:
1. starch into sugar;
2. complex sugars into absorbable forms of simple sugars such as glucose;
3. fats into fatty acids and glycerol for absorption;
4. proteins into amino acids for absorption.

(b) Absorption

These nutrients in solution are absorbed by the activity of the cells in the small intestine directly into the bloodstream and also into the small lymph vessels to the lymphatic circulation and thence to the blood for circulation to all the body cells. Water is also absorbed from the remaining bulk in the large intestine, leaving the residue for elimination as faeces on defaecation.

Activity

Draw a diagram to show how absorption occurs in the small intestine, illustrating a villus.

(c) Elimination

1 Faeces

Undigested food materials such as fibre, unabsorbed nutrients, digestive juices, bile, mucus and water are removed by defaecation. Healthy individuals vary in the amount and timing of this activity — a bowel action does not necessarily occur daily. In the healthy adult, it may be less frequent, e.g. twice weekly. In appearance, normal faeces are brown, soft in consistency, and formed.

2 Urine

This is formed by specialised cells in the kidney, whose essential function is to maintain the constant composition of the blood. One kidney is essential to maintain the life and health of the body. Waste products including the end products of protein metabolism — urea, creatinine and uric acid — pass from the blood in the 'cup' of the kidney tubule in solution into the tubule. Re-absorption into the blood capillaries of water and mineral salts, and other essential nutrients, occurs further down the loops of the kidney tubule. The solution remaining in the tubule passes from the kidney, down the ureter, to be held in the urinary bladder and voided as urine.

Normal urine is a clear amber-coloured fluid. Its specific gravity or density when compared with the density of water taken to be 1000, can be measured between 1015 and 1025 in the normal healthy person. The amount of urine voided in 24 hours by the average adult varies between 1200 and 1800 ml. N.B. Variations occur in a healthy person according to the fluid taken, and lost by other routes.

3 Sweat

Water and mineral salts are constantly being lost from the skin in the form of insensible sweat. Exercise, or an increase in the activity of the body, may increase the amount of water lost from the skin, and sweating occurs. The skin is a very important organ, with other important functions — it is protective, and a sense organ.

(d) Regulation of body temperature

The human body is a warm-blooded multicellular organism, and has to maintain its temperature within normal limits. To do so, a balance has to be achieved between heat produced in the body and heat lost from the body.

Heat is produced internally by chemical changes, particularly during digestion and muscular activity; heat may also be conducted to the body from the external environment.

Heat is lost from the body mainly through the skin (97%) in expired air during respiration (2%) and in the urine and faeces (1%). The nervous system controls the heat lost through the skin in order to keep the body in the optimum state of balance for the complex chemical changes to occur in the cells and tissues.

Movement coordination and control

The movement of the framework of the human skeleton at the joints is brought about by the action of skeletal muscles. These are sometimes called 'voluntary' muscles because they can be consciously controlled by will power. An individual can decide to lift an arm, to run or to walk. But the action of moving one limb, or two limbs, affects the balance of the individual and of his position in space. This requires coordination of the muscles elsewhere in the body, and the control within the central nervous system which is exercised on many different areas is not consciously exercised. The complexity of this control can be seen in the dexterity of the guitar player, the fine movements of a ballet dancer, athlete or trapeze artist. The equilibrium of the individual is maintained by multiple 'feedback' from joints and muscles to the spinal cord, the cerebrum and the cerebellum, as well as from the eye, the ear and the skin.

A reflex action is a movement brought about by a motor response to a sensory stimulus, e.g. dropping a hot plate.

Activity

Draw a simple diagram to illustrate a spinal reflex arc which will bring about this reflex action.

(a) Sensation

Sensation is feeling, it is the interpretation by the brain, in areas of the cortex of the cerebrum, of messages received from a network of sensory nerves carrying impulses which are generated by an end organ, or sense organ, in response to a sensory stimulus. The special sense organs, the eye, the ear, the nose, the tongue and the skin, enable the human brain to interpret the sensory messages relayed from sensory stimuli from the external environment as sight, hearing, smell, taste, touch and texture. These sensations can be life-saving; they are necessary for survival and they are essential for accuracy in making observations.

Other sensory nerve endings in joints and muscles are important in maintaining the sense of balance and in holding a pose, by enabling the brain to interpret the position of the body in space and the spatial relationships between objects.

Sensation is a very personal experience — ask two people to describe a painting, or a piece of music, and you will find examples of differing perception. The interpretation of what we see and hear is affected by memory of past experiences as well as knowledge. The sense of smell — perfume, cooking — can stimulate the memory. This is very important in nursing patients who are confused, elderly or withdrawn.

Pain

The sensation of pain in healthy individuals is a protective mechanism. Everyone has a different threshold for feeling and interpreting pain. A thorn in the finger, or a blister on the heel are painful experiences, but individuals vary in their reaction to these stimuli. Sensory nerve endings in bone, in the soft tissue of the finger or in the narrow muscular tubes (e.g. ureters) give rise to different types of pain.

Activity

List the different ways you would describe pain. What words do you use:
   (a) for toothache?
   (b) for aching muscles?
   (c) for periodic pain or dysmenorrhoea?

N.B. The nursing student needs to remember that the patient is the only person who can judge how he is affected by pain because nobody else is actually experiencing it as he does.

Reproduction

A single celled organism, such as the amoeba, or a bacterium, reproduces itself by cell division. The nucleus undergoes changes, divides itself, and then the cell protoplasm divides and two similar cells are formed.

In the human body, reproduction is bisexual. The ovum (egg cell) of the female unites with the spermatozoon (sperm cell) of the male when fertilisation occurs. A complex process then takes place concerning the chromosomes within the nucleus of each cell to form a single cell with a nucleus, the zygote. The zygote's nucleus contains 46 chromosomes — the number in every living human cell: 23 chromosomes are from the ovum, and 23 from the spermatozoon.

(a) Sex chromosomes

All ova carry two X chromosomes, which, on division of the pairs at fertilisation, from 46 to 23 chromosomes, leaves *one* X in *each* of the divisions. Sperms carry one X and one Y chromosome which, on division of the pairs at fertilisation, means there is either an X *or* a Y in each of the divisions. When the zygote results from the fertilisation of an ovum by an X chromosome sperm cell the resulting offspring is a girl, when the Y chromosome fertilises the ovum the offspring is a boy.

(b) Genes

The genes within the nucleus from the chromosomes in the male and female cell carry the inherited characteristics from generation to generation. The baby inherits these from each of his grandparents, through each of his parents. Some genes are dominant, and influence the colour of eyes and hair, and the structure of bone and height. Some are recessive.

The reproductive cycle is controlled by the balance of hormones from the gonads or sex glands. Twins and other multiple births arise from the fertilisation of more than one ovum (binovular twins) or from the fertilisation of one ovum (uniovular twins).

Further reading

DHSS, *Eating for Health,* HMSO, 1979
Jones, D., *Food for Thought,* RCN, 1975
Wilson, K., *Foundations of Anatomy and Physiology,* 5th edn (revised by Ross and Wilson), Churchill Livingstone, 1981

Suggestions for answers to Activity on page 20:
Did you consider:

noise?	overcrowding?	habits?	ignorance?
social isolation?	poverty?	peer group pressure?	loneliness?

The person

An individual's personality is unique. It is the sum total of everything about the person — the way he acts, thinks, feels, and the opinions and attitudes he holds, which may or may not be consistent with his actual behaviour. This uniqueness is in the colour of eyes, hair, skin and basic body structure, and it is expressed by his choice of clothing and belongings. The interaction between inherited, cultural and environmental influences, helps to shape the individual's personality and particular way of forming relationships with others, and making decisions about his lifestyle and practices.

The awareness a person has developed about himself, and thus the confidence he has in forming and developing relationships, depends to a large extent on his self-esteem, and how this is established and maintained.

(a) Body image and self-esteem

A newly born baby has to learn about himself and his surroundings, what is his 'self' and what is not. He starts this by exploring his body with his hands and mouth, gradually discovering where and when his body ends, and finding that he is not part of his mother, but that she is a separate, identifiable entity. This is the beginning of a learning process — the developing awareness of the body image — which brings with it the knowledge either of being the same as other people, for example, having two arms and two legs, or of being different in colour of hair, eyes, skin, yet also learning that there is a private self, which is a part of the uniqueness of the individual.

The effect on a person of discovering that he is physically different from others and is not part of the accepted 'norm', will depend to a large degree on his upbringing.

For example, a child who has no arms because his mother has taken thalidomide during her pregnancy may be overprotected by his parents, who discourage him from leading an independent life. This child may grow into adolescence unable to make friends of his own age, tending to cling to the security of home and family.

On the other hand, whilst accepting and acknowledging that such a child is different, other parents may encourage him to be adventurous, to experiment and make mistakes on the way to becoming an independent human being. This child will develop confidence in himself, in his abilities and capabilities which will help him in forming and sustaining relationships.

As the child grows and develops, he learns about himself from the feedback and cues he gets from other people, which can help to reinforce, or sometimes to damage his feelings of worthiness, of self-regard and esteem, thus affecting his confidence in the roles he adopts as he goes through life.

It can be argued that it is this growth of self-perception, that helps the individual to become aware of the feelings of others, and to be concerned for them. This is essential if meaningful relationships are to be developed and sustained. The nurse, for example, learns to put herself in the place of the patient — to share his pain, or embarrassment. She empathises with him, and is therefore able to help him adjust to a different role, to modify but maintain self-esteem.

Sometimes a person's body image may be drastically altered, for example the young man who loses a leg in a road accident. An important part of the nurse's role is to support him and his relatives during this time by helping them gradually to work through their feelings of hurt and loss. The firm but gentle way the nurse handles the young man's body, not being repulsed by the scarred limb, will help him to accept the fact that although he has lost a leg, this does not mean he is unattractive, or is less of a man.

The young married woman who has to have a breast removed must be allowed to express her grief over this loss. The nurse must accept that the woman may feel her femininity has been damaged or even lost, and may be deeply anxious about the effect of this on her husband. Will he still love me? What will the children think? are common questions asked during this period.

Both these patients must be allowed to work through their bereavement, which is the first step in the healing process. The nurse must listen with sympathy and understanding, and by her accepting manner allow the patients to express feelings of anger and frustration, without fear of rejection.

The gradual acceptance of a change in the body can be helped or marred by the reactions of others to the patients during this vulnerable period. Simple, factual, accurate explanations, and practical help in choosing a prosthesis can help the patient and the relatives to make a positive adjustment to the change in the life practices.

Definition

Prosthesis: a means of making up deficiencies, i.e. by an artificial limb, a special brassiere.

Sometimes, the patient may be unable to adapt to the change in his body; he may be afraid of the future, fearful that he will not be able to cope with his job, and what he sees as changed relationships with his loved ones. These feelings give rise to intolerable anxiety. So to escape from this conflict situation which he cannot avoid, the patient may start to regress.

Definition

Regress: to revert to a previous stage of development in which the person felt secure.

The nurse may recognise that this is happening by noticing a gradual change in the patient's behaviour, or the relatives may be the first to become aware that the patient is becoming more withdrawn, more dependent, more childish in his reactions, both emotionally and physically. The nurse and relatives must work together to treat the patient as an adult, getting him to care for himself as much as possible, gradually encouraging him to face and then to cope with reality.

Communication

The essence in any relationship is the manner in which people share their thoughts, feelings, hopes and aspirations. In other words, how they communicate with each other. The way in which the body is used, the form of dress, the facial expression, and amount and type of eye contact, as well as the tone of voice give messages to other people all the time about attitudes and feelings, as well as about social class and cultural upbringing. It is important to realise that if a person receives conflicting cues from another person communication will not be effective — there will be a block in the two-way interaction. For example, the patient hearing the nurse ask 'how are you today?' while she is anxiously watching the consultant approaching the ward, may assume that this is simply a social greeting, and respond accordingly. The nurse who sits by the bed, leans forward with an attentive manner and looks at the patient while asking the same question may receive an answer which tells her the patient is still very anxious and is in pain.

Therefore, to communicate effectively, all signals being transmitted must give the same cues so that the recipient perceives a single message. To be perceived effectively, the message must make sense to the individual. The meaning is understood when it is given in acceptable language and fits in with his previous experience.

(a) Barriers to successful communication

The nursing student should realise that patients have different perceptions about nurses; she may recognise that her patients differ in their social, cultural, economic and ethnic backgrounds — but she also needs to recognise that their

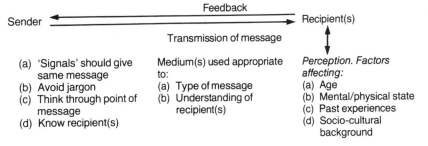

Figure 2.4   A model of communication

expectations of her own background may present a barrier to successful communication which needs to be overcome. Some may expect her to behave in a way appropriate to their perception of a nurse in interpreting their own needs and feelings, and be aggrieved if she does not realise this — others may feel her lack of understanding of their needs stems from an inability to understand because she is in a different social group, class or culture from their own.

The nurse giving information to a patient must speak in a clear voice avoiding jargon, and must ensure there is enough to obtain feedback from the patient on his understanding or otherwise. Sometimes it is better to write the information down legibly, as well as telling the patient, and his relatives. It is wise to return to the patient after time has elapsed and by careful questioning find out if his recall is still accurate.

(b) Touch

The use of touch is an essential part of communication. The person who has a limp handshake can give the immediate impression of being ineffectual. The nurse bathing a patient in bed tells him how she feels about him by the way she uses the flannel, or massages his bony prominences. A 'scrubbing action' used in either, can communicate lack of interest and boredom to the patient, as well as losing him some essential thicknesses of skin!

(c) Dexterity

An essentially practical skill, like removing sutures from a wound, is broken down into smaller components for teaching/learning purposes. The student is encouraged to practise the handling of forceps, to inject water into an orange, because clumsiness is not only potentially dangerous, but can give the patient further pain and discomfort, and destroy his trust in the nurse.

Groups

It is in communication with others that an individual gets feedback about himself, and it is in his relationships with others he fulfils his needs to share and belong, to participate and to love.

This does not mean that a person needs to spend all his waking hours in the company of others. Individuals also need time to themselves, to think and reflect, to listen and read and write, and to be alone.

From the moment of conception, there is interaction between two organisms, the mother and the foetus, which continues during pregnancy and after the child is born. The unborn child gives evidence of his presence by the movements he makes.

The mother can affect the unborn child by the choices she makes about her own life. For example, if she smokes constantly and heavily during pregnancy the baby may be born smaller than the norm, less resistant to infections.

This interaction, the relationship which develops between mother and child, child with father and siblings, and later with peer groups, is essential for growth and development. It is with others that a person can share his thoughts and feelings, hopes and aspirations.

Two or more people together form a group, and groups can be large or small. The aims of the group will differ according to the needs of the individuals making up the group, and the reasons why the group has formed.

The smaller the group, the more face to face contact and communication, and intimate relationships can develop in an informal atmosphere.

The larger the group, the more formal will the structure become, and communications will take place through an intermediary or intermediaries such as another person, or by written or telephoned messages.

Receiving information by indirect means can result in misunderstandings and misconceptions as an individual cannot ask directly for clarification, and does not receive other clues to help him in his understanding.

The infant is born into his family or primary group where relationships are informal and the language is meaningful to all members. The customs and practices of the family are determined by the culture, and the social class structure into which the child is born.

The values and standards of conduct practised by the family will, to a greater or lesser extent, influence the individual throughout his life, acting as a yard-stick or reference upon which to base his own opinions, decisions and behaviour.

The child of Bengali parents born in the East End of London will grow up among relatives and friends who speak his parents' language and follow similar racial customs, but outside these groups he will probably have to work and play with others, such as white English people, or black West Indians who may speak a different language, eat different food, worship God differently. These 'significant others' may exhibit a closeness and cohesiveness in their groups which prevents him from becoming a member, or even if he is made a formal member because of being in the same work and workplace, they make him feel unwanted by their reactions.

As the child grows and matures he participates in many, and different, groups, sometimes becoming a member of a smaller group within a larger setting. For example, in the formal classroom group he receives instruction from the formal leader, the teacher, but he and his friends form social groups in the playground and outside school. The accepted leader of the gang may be the most dominant, or the most respected, or the most liked or feared, but often another child will become the leader for a specific occasion when his particular skills are required by the others. For example, the child who knows the route through the fence to the farmer's orchard to 'scrump' apples leads the way!

Nursing students form a group when they enter nursing. The main aim is to become a qualified nurse, but another aim may be to work together as a group to make their views on patient care known to their teachers or to the nursing manager. Within the main group, sub-groups develop, for example, friendship groups, individuals coming together only for study purposes, or to play tennis, and so on. At the same time, the nursing student remains a member of her family and other groups, and also becomes a member of the health care team for a short period of time. She is daughter, and girl friend, the chairman of the tennis club, a member of a political party, as well as a nursing student.

In each group, the members decide upon certain standards of behaviour to which each individual is expected to conform. In formal groups, such as the nursing profession itself, or within the school of nursing, or the health care team, these become rules and regulations. If a member does not wish to conform, he can leave, or comply while he is within the particular group, or endeavour to modify or change the expectations of the group. The influence an individual exerts depends on his role and status within the group and how he is accepted by the other members. For example, the ward sister/charge nurse/district nurse is the accepted formal leader in the nursing team, with authority invested in her because of her role. She makes decisions and accepts responsibility for the patients and nursing students in her charge.

Activity

Here is a list of roles which may be adopted by an individual. Write down the behaviour you think will be exhibited by the person in that particular role. Why do you think the person has adopted that role? Discuss with your colleagues and teacher.

Perhaps you can think of other roles not mentioned here.

Leader	Follower
Second in command	Mediator
Scapegoat	Comforter
Joker	'Stirrer'

Roles

As the infant grows and matures physically, emotionally and intellectually he learns to adapt to different environments, like going to school instead of being at home. He also starts to meet many more people. From birth until the age of about five, his mother, father, siblings and other relatives have been the prime focus of his world, the people with whom he identifies. At school he mingles with peers, forms gangs and learns to conform to what is expected of him by his friends and teachers. In other words he becomes a member of different groups and starts to adopt many different roles as he develops from baby to 'toddler', to child at school, adolescent starting work, young man starting to date, to marrying, eventually leading to retirement and death. At any time this cycle can be interrupted by sickness, when for a time the responsibility of satisfying his own needs may be undertaken by others.

A person adopts many different roles at the same time, the predominant one at any given time being adopted according to the particular circumstances. For example Mr Smith aged 50, the breadwinner of his family, a stalwart member of his church, and a leading bridge player, adopts the role and behaviour of a patient when sick and in hospital; this behaviour is very different from his normal lifestyle.

Definition

A role can be defined as the part one plays, and with it can come status in the eyes of others, as well as confidence for the individual, by boosting his self-esteem.

Role and behaviour

The particular behaviour one adopts as a son or daughter, may be different from the way one behaves as the leader of a tennis team, or as a patient, or as a nurse, or a nursing student.

Sometimes a certain type of behaviour becomes expected from an individual in a particular role, and this 'stereotyping' can have both beneficial and adverse effects. For example, the image of a patient is often one who is dependent, passive and thankful. Much anxiety can be felt among nurses, doctors, and indeed relatives, if the patient becomes vocal, aggressively demanding to know what medicines or treatment are being prescribed and why. When the patient claims, firmly and rightly, that he has the right to know what is being done to his own body, this may cause mixed feelings of doubt and righteousness among 'the carers'.

The first year nursing student can increase her confidence and assurance by wearing a uniform when attending to patients, who respond as if they consider she is kind, sympathetic and skilled. The student's behaviour produced by this 'patient response' is often that which is expected by the patient, this therefore confirms the patient's expectations of the nurse in her role. The patient views the nurse as a safe person, and sometimes displaces his fear and anxieties in the form of aggression on to the nurse, because she is seen as secure. The young student has to learn to cope with these displaced feelings of the patient, which takes time and knowledge, plus help and support from qualified nurses. She has to learn that it is not herself, i.e. as Jane the daughter, who is the cause of this anger, but student nurse Jones who is expected by the patient to understand, to remain unchanged and undamaged and to cope with the situation.

The learner has to appreciate that there are many aspects to her role as a nursing student. To the patients, she is capable and confident, to the doctors and other members of the caring team she is a colleague with particular expertise, to the tutor she is someone who needs support while learning, and to the ward sister she is someone who requires supervision much of the time. It is no wonder that nursing is seen as a demanding, albeit rewarding profession!!

Learning

Those learning to nurse have to give care to patients/clients which is emotionally and physically demanding, and at the same time to acquire the knowledge which is essential to the skilled performance in the giving of this care. As the student currently spends approximately 65% of her time in the clinical setting, this is where much of learning occurs. The student will learn by observing how the other members of the nursing team, the enrolled or registered nurses, the staff nurse, sister or teacher relate to patients, relatives and others. Particular behaviours and attitudes which are found to be acceptable and desirable will be 'internalised' by the student and become part of her own system of values and beliefs. For example, the best way a student can learn how to cope with bereaved relatives is to take part with sister in their comforting. This way she will learn that it is sometimes desirable for a nurse to express her feelings by crying with others, and that this is normal and acceptable behaviour. She will learn how to listen in silence and how to answer questions of doubts, fears and feelings of relief or guilt.

It is essential that the student has time away from the wards to be with her colleagues to share experiences, and for her learning to be deepened and consolidated. Study sessions are arranged by the teachers of nursing, who plan programmes of study which enable the student to develop and deepen her perceptions of nursing and nursing practices. Teaching sessions are organised in teaching rooms and clinical areas, with the teachers acting the role of the tutor, facilitator or counsellor according to the needs of the student. The student learns that the lecture is only one method of gaining information; that self-directed learning which is helped and guided by the tutor can be exciting and rewarding, as well as long lasting. The more active a student is in pursuing, applying and adapting knowledge, the more meaningful and relevant it becomes in her role as a nurse. Reasoning and adapting become part of the normal process of the giving of individualised patient care. The nursing student learns how to assess the patient's needs in priority order, how to plan and carry out effective care, and at all times learns to look at her own performance with a critical eye, so that her future care can be modified or changed for the benefit of the patient.

At the beginning of nursing training, the student may find that being involved with patients and their relatives and living in the hospital environment can be overwhelming and excluding. It is essential for her mental, social and physical health that the student maintains her social contacts, going out with friends, and pursuing her usual hobbies and interests. Sometimes the very involvement with patients and colleagues which nursing entails can become so absorbing that the ability to stand aside to be reflective and objective, is lost. The student can become drained of energy, or her anxiety may become overwhelming. It is the responsibility of the teacher, the trained nurse and the student's colleagues to recognise that this is happening, and to provide the support and seek the sources of expert help which are needed to aid the student to come to terms with the problem.

The Health Care Team

The student has to learn that giving care to patients/clients is not the sole province of the nurse, that others are essential as part of a professional health team who work together for the benefit of the patients. The patient and his relatives are central and should participate. They have certain rights and privileges which must be respected. The student and trained nurse are important persons in this caring team, who take responsibility for their actions in helping the patient to recover his usual health, in assisting him to live with disability, or by helping him to a dignified death.

The main aim of the health care team is to enable the patient to remain in and to resume his place in the community, either by restoring him to his usual health, or by assisting him to cope with disablement or disability.

The members of this team involved in the patient/client's care may include the doctor, the social worker, the physiotherapist, the occupational therapist, the dietician, as well as the nurse. An important member of the nursing team is the nursing auxiliary, who can provide a constant, unchanging stable element to the team. The different chaplains play an important part in the welfare of the patient by providing a counselling as well as a spiritual service not only to patients, and their relatives, but also to staff members.

Each member of the team is concerned with the ongoing assessment and management of the patient, and they work together by pooling their specialist knowledge, and by complementing each other's expertise and actions. This expertise, which enables each member to fill a particular role, is developed through a specific training course, which is controlled by a statutory or non-statutory body, and for which particular entrance qualifications are required. There are many overlapping functions, however, in each particular team member's role, and there must be frequent ongoing discussions between them, and with the patient and his relatives to ensure that safe and relevant practices are achieved.

The team members either work mainly in the hospital, *or* in the community, so effective communication between colleagues is essential to maintain the continuum of patient care from hospital to home or vice versa. The professional team is assisted in its work by members of many voluntary agencies, such as The British Red Cross Society, St John's Ambulance Brigade, and the National Association of Mental Health (MIND). Volunteers from these organisations may work with patients, perform simple practical tasks like hair washing, and listening to anxieties or reminiscences with understanding and empathy. In the care of the long term chronic sick in institutions, the volunteer can provide a link with the outside world. Charities like MIND also run homes and hostels for disturbed children, adolescents and adults, as well as organising courses on mental health, and acting as a pressure group to influence government in its treatment of the mentally ill.

The doctor's main function is to diagnose and prescribe the appropriate medical treatment for the patient. This treatment is often carried out by the nurse, who also assesses the nursing needs of the patient. The planning, carrying out and the evaluation of this care must involve the patient and his relatives, and forms a major part of the role of the nurse. A senior nurse may also plan the care according to need for a group of patients in her charge. In the community much of the work of the doctor and nurse is geared to the maintenance and promotion of health, and the prevention of ill health. Nurses in the community have further specialist training to prepare them for this work.

The district nurse plans, carries out and assesses the effectiveness of her nursing care of a person at home, often providing an essential link between the individual and the outside world. She often works closely with community psychiatric nurses who help the individual and his relatives cope with stresses which have affected the person's mental health.

The health visitor liaises closely with the doctor, district nurse and social worker to ensure the client knows which services are appropriate and available, and to assist him to make decisions about his life practices; for example, suggesting and giving practical help on family planning to the husband and wife who decide not to have any more children.

The health visitor and social worker observe clients in their homes, and help both the person and the relatives to identify needs and to cope themselves, or with help, with their problems and stresses of living. The health visitor and social worker develop a special knowledge of their client's socio-economic background, and an awareness of the particular family relationships, which helps them to fulfil their role.

The midwife helps the pregnant mother by skilled antenatal care to ensure that complications such as inappropriately high blood pressure, which can adversely affect both mother and unborn child, are recognised or avoided. The midwife can actually assist the mother to cut down smoking, alcohol consumption, or excess food, if the mother decides that this is what she wants to do. It is in the helping of the mother to come to this decision that special knowledge plus an ability to communicate a non-judgmental attitude is essential. The midwife also delivers the baby in the hospital, or in the home, using her special expertise to know when to call for the assistance of the doctor or emergency squad to avoid prolonged or harmful labour.

The after care of the mother and child is shared by the midwife and the health visitor who, together, aid the family with practical instruction, for example, on breast feeding, bathing the baby, and with advice on an immunisation programme.

The physiotherapist and occupational therapist both work with the patient by himself, or with other patients forming a group. They assess the patient's actual performance, and potential for development, and help the patient achieve the maximum use possible of his body and mind.

For example, the physiotherapist can help the patient use a partially paralysed arm by encouraging him to exercise regularly using a particular technique. The occupational therapist can encourage this by getting an adaption made to everyday equipment, like a special large handle to a spoon or knife to aid grip. The occupational therapist and physiotherapist work together to enable the individual to achieve maximum independence in activities needed for daily living, e.g. in cooking, housework, gardening, as well as helping the person enjoy unsuspected talents, for example, in painting or knitting.

The body interacts with and is dependent on the 'mind' and vice versa, so that the gradual mastery of simple motor skills can give pleasure, and perhaps emotional relief, as well as helping a partially paralysed individual adjust to a change in body image, as well as maintaining his self-esteem.

Food is important to all individuals, whatever their cultural background, and when a person becomes ill it is vital that he maintains adequate appropriate nourishment to maintain his body functions. The dietician works through the catering department and with the doctor and nurse to ensure that the individual's dietary requirements for health, and for the change brought about by disease, are worked out accurately, with due regard to the amount and type and to the person's preferences, and religious or cultural background. The dietician must therefore have frequent contact with her patients, or clients, and with the nurses, to see if the food is, in fact, being eaten, and if so, if it is eaten reluctantly or with relish.

There are other professionals and staff who contribute to the care and management of the patient in hospital, and client in the community.

The clinical psychologist is largely concerned with the understanding of behaviour in relation to illness, and offers a contribution to the objective assessment of an individual's performance and potential by interpreting the results from a battery of tests.

The administrator in the hospital co-ordinates the various groups of workers and helps to ensure the smooth everyday running of the institution.

The receptionist in the clinic or ward can influence the individual's attitude to treatment by the manner which she employs to greet the patient. A pleasant smile and soothing voice together with accurate information can do much to help allay fears and anxieties.

The members of the team who provide treatment and support for the individual are responsible to, and for, the individual in their care. The trained people are also accountable for their actions in the carrying out of particular treatments and care. Accountable not just legally, but also to their colleagues with whom they share responsibility, and to the patient/client and his relatives who depend on their expert services.

The care study given below will illustrate the way certain individuals and groups work together and with the patient, to allow him to achieve optimum health and independence.

Care study

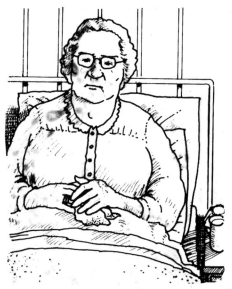

Figure 2.5   Mrs Green

Mrs Green, aged 75, a widow living alone in a high rise flat, was admitted to hospital for further investigations and treatment of her diabetes mellitus. On admission to the ward, her condition was described as 'unstable', meaning that her diabetes was not being controlled adequately.

The nurse admitted Mrs Green to the ward, and assessed her needs, in priority order.

For example, Mrs Green was a large lady, so she was sitting upright in bed to allow her to breathe more easily, and to enable her to cough and expectorate, which she did frequently. This was encouraged by the nurse and physiotherapist, as it would keep the lungs clear, and help prevent patchy collapse of lung tissue.

The doctor examined Mrs Green thoroughly, and ordered investigations to be carried out by the technicians in the haematology department. For example, blood was examined to detect if the blood glucose level was higher than normal for Mrs Green.

After the investigations and the results were received, the doctor ordered a special diet for Mrs Green, low in calories and carbohydrate. He also ordered

REGIONAL AND DISTRICT HEALTH AUTHORITIES, AND FAMILY PRACTITIONER COMMITTEES

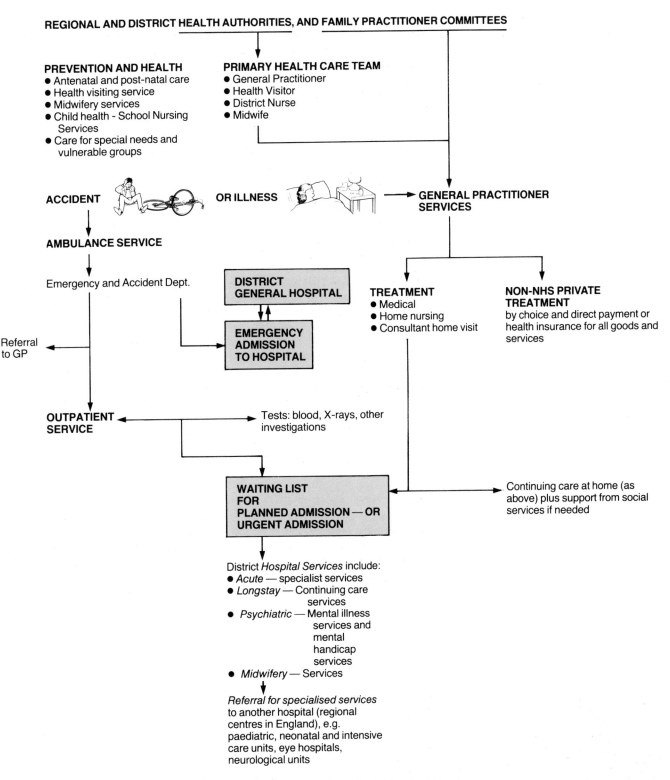

PREVENTION AND HEALTH
- Antenatal and post-natal care
- Health visiting service
- Midwifery services
- Child health - School Nursing Services
- Care for special needs and vulnerable groups

PRIMARY HEALTH CARE TEAM
- General Practitioner
- Health Visitor
- District Nurse
- Midwife

ACCIDENT   **OR ILLNESS**   **GENERAL PRACTITIONER SERVICES**

AMBULANCE SERVICE

Emergency and Accident Dept.

DISTRICT GENERAL HOSPITAL

EMERGENCY ADMISSION TO HOSPITAL

Referral to GP

TREATMENT
- Medical
- Home nursing
- Consultant home visit

NON-NHS PRIVATE TREATMENT
by choice and direct payment or health insurance for all goods and services

OUTPATIENT SERVICE

Tests: blood, X-rays, other investigations

Continuing care at home (as above) plus support from social services if needed

WAITING LIST FOR PLANNED ADMISSION — OR URGENT ADMISSION

District *Hospital Services* include:
- *Acute* — specialist services
- *Longstay* — Continuing care services
- *Psychiatric* — Mental illness services and mental handicap services
- *Midwifery* — Services

Referral for specialised services to another hospital (regional centres in England), e.g. paediatric, neonatal and intensive care units, eye hospitals, neurological units

Figure 2.6   The National Health Service in England
Under the National Health Service, either at home or in hospital, all treatment, medicines, goods and services are provided free at the point of delivery for all — except dental care, opticians' costs, prescription charges (i.e. not the full cost of the medication).
These exceptions are, however, not charged for vulnerable groups, e.g. children, pregnant women, and those requiring permanent medication.
Individuals choosing to pay fees for private medical treatment and nursing care, pay the full cost of their medication and appliances, and pay for any access to National Health Service departments for investigation and treatment

tablets for her to take which would stimulate cells in her body to produce more insulin to help the utilisation of the glucose. The nurses made sure that the correct tablets were swallowed by Mrs Green at the right time of day.

The dietician visited Mrs Green to ask her what foods she liked, and to work out a diet which would be acceptable to her which included the correct nutrients in the right amounts.

Both the dietician and nurse talked frequently with Mrs Green, and her only relative, a niece, to ensure the importance of eating the food at the correct times was understood. Opportunity was taken to listen to any queries, and to find out about Mrs Green's home circumstances. The domestic in the ward also made time to chat when taking around the tea trolley — an important time for socialisation.

The chiropodist was asked to visit Mrs Green, and with her consent, trimmed her toe-nails, which were horny and overgrown, and removed hard skin from the soles of her feet. The chiropodist used his expertise to make sure no skin areas were cut, as infection was more likely to occur because of Mrs Green's diabetic condition. The nurse ensured that Mrs Green's feet were always washed, and dried very thoroughly. The reason for this was carefully explained to Mrs Green and her niece.

During her stay in the ward, Mrs Green chose library books in big print, from the trolley wheeled around and kept stocked by volunteers from The League of Friends.

The day before Mrs Green was ready for discharge, her GP and the Community Nursing Service were alerted and given full details of her admission and care. The health visitor had continued to visit her while she was in hospital.

It was arranged that the district nurse would visit her daily, and arrange help for Mrs Green to bath herself, as was her normal practice. The district nurse liaised closely with Mrs Green's own doctor, the health visitor and her niece who lived nearby.

Home-help service was provided, so that Mrs Green had her flat cleaned thoroughly twice a week. The home-help also did all the shopping, and knew whom to contact should assistance be needed.

The social worker was contacted to see if any pressure could be brought on to the housing department to enable Mrs Green to move to a ground floor flat, with easy access to shops and parks.

The laundry service arranged for dirty sheets to be collected and provided clean bed linen once a week. Mrs Green's niece and the home-help encouraged her to wash her own clothes, to retain as much independence as possible.

The meals on wheels service could have provided the special diet, but it was agreed by Mrs Green, her niece and the district nurse that Mrs Green herself would be able to cook her own food, and follow her diet sheet correctly. She knew that she could always ask the district nurse, or the health visitor who called round, for help and advice.

Mrs Green had an appointment arranged to return to the hospital to see the doctor, and she travelled sitting in an ambulance along with other people who also had to attend. The ambulance man made sure they were sitting comfortably.

The local British Red Cross Society arranged with the district nurse that a member should visit Mrs Green weekly, to chat with her and to keep her company, and to help her wash her hair once a fortnight.

Mrs Green gradually returned to her usual lifestyle, which included a weekly visit to the local 'Darby and Joan' Club for company, and to indulge in the weekly bingo session. She also visited her local public house for her weekly half pint of Guinness, which she thoroughly enjoyed as she shared gossip with her friends.

References

Disraeli, B., A speech made in Battersea Park on June 23rd, 1877 and reported in *The Times,* June 25th, 1877

Jay, P., *Report of the Committee of Enquiry into Mental Handicap and Nursing Care,* HMSO, 1978

Mansfield, K., *Letters and Journals,* Penguin, 1977

Warnock, M., Special Educational Needs — Report of the Committee of Enquiry into the Education of Handicapped Children and Young People, Cmnd, 7212, 1978

WHO, *World Health Organization Constitution,* WHO, Geneva, 1947

Further reading

Altschul, A. and Sinclair, H., *Psychology for Nurses,* 5th edn, Baillière Tindall, 1981

Collins, M., *Communication in Health Care,* C. V. Mosby Co., 1977

Davies, B., *Community Health, Preventive Medicine and Social Services,* Meredith, 1981

Hilgard, E. R., Atkinson, R. L. and Atkinson, R. C., *Introduction to Psychology,* 7th edn, Harcourt Brace Jovanovich, 1979

James, D. E., *Introduction to Psychology,* Constable, 1970

Jasmin, S. and Tygstad, L. N., *Behavioural Concepts and the Nursing Process,* C. V. Mosby Co., 1979

McGhee, A., *Psychology as Applied to Nursing,* 7th edn, Churchill Livingstone, 1979

Shafer, K.N., Sawyer, J.R., McCluskey, A., Beck, E.L. and Phipps, W.J., *Medical and Surgical Nursing,* 6th edn, C.V. Mosby Co., 1975.

Sprott, W. J. H., *Human Groups,* Pelican Books, 1969

Chapter 3   Illness

The external environment in illness

The human body in health can modify its activities to respond to changes in the external environment, and to keep the internal environment in balance under different circumstances; for example, in the healthy individual as the day becomes hotter, the amount of sweat lost from the skin increases and blood vessels in the skin are dilated to supply more blood to the sweat glands and the skin colour is increased; in cold weather, the skin appears pale because the converse has occurred to maintain the body temperature.

The safety of the body can be assisted in extremely cold conditions by more warm clothing, by food, by movement, by conserving the heat of the body by using a plastic bag, as when exposed on a mountain side in adverse weather conditions.

In ordinary everyday life, the healthy person can avoid hazards in the external environment to preserve his safety. Most people learn to avoid such hazards for their own comfort. The baby learning to crawl and the toddler learning to climb need other people to check the safety of their surroundings. The nurse has to learn to modify the environment for a person who has a disability — whose movement is under strain or limited — and for a person who is ill and whose surroundings are new to him. The adult who is attending an out-patient clinic, or who has arrived at the Admissions Office of a hospital on receipt of a letter, is now a patient — the environment is different — he needs cues and direct information to proceed with day-to-day activities.

Preventing the hazards of illness

Florence Nightingale (1859) said that 'The hospital should do the patient no harm'; wherever the nurse works, this should be remembered.

(a) Fire

It is vital that every member of the nursing staff in a clinic or hospital should have detailed knowledge of the procedure to be followed in the event of an outbreak of fire. Patients' lives are at risk from asphyxia due to smoke as well as from the effect of burns caused by flames. The nurse should report a suspected outbreak at once and take simple first aid measures, such as damp cloths over the mouth and nose, and the immediate removal of all those who can move, from the vicinity of the smoke and fire. There are fire officers in each health district in the UK who advise, and teach about measures for preventing fire as well as those to be taken for a suspected outbreak.

(b) Flooding

In some centres there is also a risk of flooding, and where this is possible there will be a procedure to be followed which every nursing student also needs to learn.

Activity

1. List the regulations for 'fire prevention' in your own nursing school and the 'procedure to be undertaken in case of flooding'.
2. List the factors which will prevent people responding to a fire alarm.

Other local hazards such as the escape of noxious chemical fumes from industrial plants, or the discharge of chemical material into rivers, polluting water supplies, are the concern of environmental health officers who give advice on special measures in such circumstances.

(c) Radiation

Hospitals use radium and other radioactive materials for the treatment of malignant disease, and for routine tests on blood chemistry and bodily activity. These are used under strict control and there are special rules for all those coming into contact with them during use. The physicist and the radiotherapist will be responsible, with the help of medical and nursing staff, for providing these rules for safe practice. Radiation detection badges are worn by staff for their protection in clinics, wards and operating theatres where radiotherapy takes place.

(d) Poisons

Poisonous substances are used as household cleaning agents and in the investigation and treatment of disease. In the laboratories, technicians and medical staff are required to observe strict rules for their care, storage and use. In the wards and departments of the hospital where medicines are given according to the doctor's prescription for the patient, there are strict rules also for their use and their custody. The chief pharmacist is legally held responsible for the amount and use of controlled drugs in hospital. He and his assistants are available for advice regarding the use and care of all medicines in the hospital.

Storage, safe custody and giving of medicines in hospital wards, departments and clinics

(a) The legislation in the United Kingdom

1   The Misuse of Drugs Act 1971

This sets out government regulations regarding the ordering, custody and administration of drugs to which a person may become habituated, e.g. pethidine, morphine, heroin.

2   The Medicines (Prescription Only) Order 1977

This lists drugs which, because of their action and side effects, must be prescribed by a doctor, e.g. diazepam.

3   The Medicines (General Sales List) Order 1977

This lists drugs which may be bought by the general public without a doctor's prescription, e.g. aspirin.

(b) The ordering of medicines

The pharmacy supplies medicines to be used in wards and departments of a hospital on the receipt of an appropriate written order. This may be either a written prescription authorised and signed by a doctor, or it may be a requisition form signed by a registered nurse. When medicines are delivered to the ward, they should be received, checked and put away immediately in a locked cupboard, according to their type. Those medications prescribed for external use, e.g. creams or lotions, should be kept in a separate locked cupboard, fluids for intravenous infusion in another place, and those for internal use in a locked cupboard or locked trolley for administration.

Definition

Intravenous: into a vein.

(c) The care of medicines

Controlled drugs (those to which a person may become habituated) must be kept in a specially labelled and locked cupboard within another locked cupboard. The amount of these drugs in stock in the cupboard should be checked and counted daily, and also counted, checked and noted after a drug has been used. Any discrepancy in this record should be reported at once to a nursing officer and the pharmacist so that further enquiries can be made. The sister or charge nurse in the ward is responsible for the custody and the use of these drugs in the ward and is answerable for their care to the pharmacist who is responsible for the total amount used within the hospital.

Medicines and drugs are ordered for use and to be given as prescribed by a doctor to a patient. They may not be given to anyone else, e.g. to a visitor or a member of staff.

The misuse of medicines and drugs — and therefore of her professional knowledge, is a form of professional misconduct for which a qualified nurse may be called to account by the statutory body (see page 6).

(d) The giving of medicines

Wherever a medicine is prescribed for a patient by a doctor great care should be taken that the patient, the relative if the patient is at home, and the nurse know the *time* at which it is to be taken, and the *amount* that is to be taken, and the way in which it is to be taken.

There are different routes for substances to be taken for different actions. They can, for example, be:

Inhaled — as a medication or during an anaesthetic.
Swallowed — to be absorbed in the gastrointestinal tract.
Applied to the skin — lotions and creams.
Dropped into the nose, the ears or the eyes.
Injected by syringe and needle:
  into the layers of the skin — intradermal;
  into the tissue below the skin — subcutaneous;
  into the muscle below the skin — intramuscular;
  into the vein, therefore directly to the blood — intravenously;
  into the body cavities, e.g. the peritoneal or pleural cavities, or the theca (the subarachnoid space).

Accuracy in giving medication to patients is essential — particularly when the nurse may be caring for several patients or when several nurses in a team are caring for one patient. A clearly written record that a medicine has been given should be made immediately to avoid mistakes. Patients in hospital wear a wrist band, or identity bracelet, and before giving any medication the nurse should check the written prescription, the label on the container, and the wrist band to identify that the correct procedure is being followed.

If any mistake should occur, either an error in the calculation of the amount of the drug measured, or if the medicine is given at the wrong time, or to the wrong patient, prompt reporting of the error enables the appropriate remedial action to be taken by the nursing and medical staff. It is very important to try to prevent errors by following the agreed procedures correctly — *it may be life-saving, however, to report when any possible mistake may have been made.*

Activity

List and consider the methods used in your own training school to ensure the safety of the patient when medicines are:

- ordered from pharmacy;
- prescribed by a doctor;
- given by a nurse.

Body defences

The individual has a mind, body and soul which are interrelated and function together making a complete whole.

Disturbance of the 'norm' for the individual, caused by internal and/or external factors may produce signs and symptoms which alert the person, or others, that something is wrong. For example, the individual with acute food poisoning may vomit, a sign of gastric upset which also serves as a protective mechanism by helping to excrete the pathogenic organisms, or the widow who has recently lost a beloved husband may weep frequently and at unexpected times.

Anxiety is an emotion closely allied to fear. It can be caused by external events such as the threat of warfare, or by interactions with others which cause a lowering of, or damage to, the individual's self-esteem. For example, the patient may feel depersonalised in hospital because the nurses and doctors treat him as an object, and not as an individual. Volicer and Bohammon (1975) examined aspects of hospital life which were perceived as stressful to patients. They found that problems relating to sleeping or eating were less stressful than a lack of information, or meaningful communication from hospital staff. In some circumstances, however, an increase in anxiety can act as a motivating force. For example, the realisation that an examination is looming may stimulate the person to further study.

In situations which produce anxiety, e.g. when confronted by a rabid dog, the autonomic nervous system is motivated, and glands in the body secrete more hormones, adrenaline and noradrenaline, which affect certain organs in the body. The result is that the person can run away quickly out of danger because the heart beats faster, arterial pressure rises, and there is more blood, oxygen and glucose supplied to vital organs such as the muscles, heart and brain. The bronchial tubes in the lungs relax so that breathing is easier. The pupils of the eyes dilate so that the danger can be seen. This is sometimes known as the fright, fight and flight mechanism.

Emotional or psychological stresses play a large part in the causation of certain illnesses in which physical symptoms appear to be predominant. These illnesses are often labelled 'psychosomatic'. In bronchial asthma, the bronchioles in the lungs go into spasm causing the person to have difficulty in breathing, particularly in breathing out. The cause of the attack may be bronchial infection, an allergy to cat's fur, severe stress, or be unknown or a mixture of factors.

Example: A child may have a bronchial asthma attack whenever he hears and/or sees, his parents quarrelling.

In situations which cause stress to the individual, anxiety increases and defence mechanisms in the body become activated to prevent, or lessen damage. Sometimes these responses may become maladaptive, or pathological, causing harm.

Coping strategies: personality defence mechanisms

Personality defence mechanisms exist in everyone to a lesser or greater degree. In the normal way they help the individual cope with anxiety, to protect him from feeling inadequate thus enabling his own idea of himself, his self-esteem, to be preserved. These mechanisms operate at an unconscious level so that the individual at the time is not aware of what is happening, although others who know the person well may become aware of the situation by accurate observation.

(a) Regression

This has already been mentioned in the text, and is an example of these personality defence mechanisms. An individual regresses to a previous secure stage in his development to 'avoid' the current situation which is causing anxiety. An elderly patient in a regressed state will appear more childish, more dependent, often with physical deterioration occurring, and urinating in the bed or in his clothes. When the ward where elderly patients are cared for is very busy, and there is a shortage of staff, the nurses may encourage regression in their patients by doing everything for them, because it is quicker and easier. The policy of care in a ward or home which has long-term elderly patients must include the prevention of regression by strategies such as reality orientation programmes. Here the patients/clients are addressed by the name they wish others to use, dress themselves in their own clothes, have the date and day in big letters on the wall, and daily news events are discussed. All means are taken to encourage the patients to be aware of and live in the present, real situation.

Regression can be transient, as happens when John, aged five, reverts to thumb-sucking and bed-wetting when his baby sister is born. Mother and father realise that John is feeling lost and bewildered, perhaps jealous of the attention his sister is receiving, and give him a lot of love and attention by cuddling him and including him in all that is happening.

(b) Repression

Unacceptable thoughts, feelings, impulses which cause guilt and are unacceptable to the individual are repressed, that is 'removed' from the conscious awareness.

During a lifespan, a person sometimes behaves in a way he often regrets. If the memory of this were always present in his thoughts, life would be intolerable, therefore repression occurs to help him function normally. For example, the middle-aged mother does not recall hitting her baby son whenever he was naughty.

(c) Rationalisation

This refers to the process of giving logical, acceptable reasons for one's behaviour. The nursing student for example, might say, and believe, that the reason she did not pass the examination was because at the time she had a severe headache. The unacceptable truth is that she did not study for the examination, and could not answer the questions.

The patient may say that she forgot to tell the doctor about some distressing symptoms. The real reason, however, is that she is afraid to discover what she fears is the real diagnosis.

(d) Introjection

This occurs when qualities, ideals seen as desirable possessed by another admired person or object are internalised into the individual's own value system, becoming part of his personality. This can occur during childhood when the infant identifies with his parents, the son becoming a miniature of his father with similar values and attitudes. Sometimes this leads to socially unacceptable behaviour; for example, if the father is a thief and believes this is the right way of living. On the other hand the student nurse may incorporate the beliefs and ideals of the nursing profession into her own value system as she learns from nurses she respects and admires.

(e) Projection

This is the opposite of introjection. Qualities, traits in an individual which are unacceptable are denied and attributed to others. The student nurse may complain that a patient does not like her, because her own feelings of dislike for the patient cause guilt and anxiety. The nursing student who feels a patient dislikes her will react to the patient accordingly, and the patient may respond with behaviour which reinforces the student's feelings — a self-fulfilling prophecy which is not beneficial to the participants' well-being. It is important that nursing students accept that they will not automatically like every patient. In the discussions on patient care held daily in the ward, the expression of feelings about the patients should be encouraged, so that the reasons can be explored, and ways and means developed to help the nurse and the nursing student to cope in her relationship with the patient.

(f) Sublimation

This occurs when repressed urges are directed into socially approved channels. The lonely, elderly widow may gratify her need for love and affection by adopting and caring for stray animals, or becoming involved with the League of Friends at the local children's hospital.

Non-coping strategies

Sometimes these personality or ego defence mechanisms become maladaptive. For example, *denial* occurs when the patient believes he is going to recover and go back to his normal employment when in reality he is not going to get well again and this has been fully explained.

Some situations produce severe anxiety with which the individual is unable to cope, and he becomes mentally ill; for example, with an acute, or chronic anxiety state in which physical symptoms often predominate. The person may complain of tenseness, headache, and palpitations as well as feeling very anxious and worried. Often the individual cannot pinpoint what is specifically causing his anxiety, so it is called 'free-floating' anxiety.

Physical responses

The individual in a state of shock due to physical injury and/or emotional trauma looks pale, feels cold to the touch and may faint. The reason for this is that the superficial blood vessels have constricted, enabling more blood to circulate to essential internal organs. Fainting is a protective mechanism because it enables the heart to pump blood to the brain more effectively.

In shock due to pain and excess blood loss, for example, the loss of a limb in an accident, or the erosion of a blood vessel in the lining of the stomach due to an ulcer, the production of red blood corpuscles which carry oxygen is increased, and the blood pressure in the body is maintained by substances being released by the kidneys, which respond to a sustained shortage of oxygen.

In times of prolonged shock, e.g. someone who is severely burned, and also in starvation, the body reacts by causing the cells in the liver to reconvert glycogen to glucose which can be used to maintain heat and energy. Other hormones produced in the body, for example cortisol from the adrenal glands, also help in this reaction.

External/internal body defences

There are other defence mechanisms which normally operate in the body and are essential to the individual's survival. The person is at risk if the mechanisms malfunction or are non-existent. For example, the baby born with inadequate bone marrow which is not producing special cells (antibodies) is at risk from infections.

Micro-organisms need specific conditions, for example, the correct chemical environment, to grow and multiply. The human body produces different secretions which may be alkaline or acid, which allow the growth of some organisms, but kill others. The highly acid secretions produced by special cells in the lining of the stomach kill many of the organisms eaten with food. Other organisms, like those that cause food poisoning, can exist until they arrive in the large intestine which provides the right conditions for growth. Here the organisms reproduce rapidly and by this action cause the symptoms of acute gastrointestinal upset, diarrhoea and vomiting. These symptoms alert the individual and others that something is wrong, and also help to excrete the pathogenic organisms quickly.

Vaginal secretions contain acid, which kills most pathogenic organisms entering the vagina, except for the organisms causing syphilis and gonorrhoea. Vaginal secretions are not present before puberty and are decreased following the menopause. The young girl and the older woman are therefore at particular risk, and should be taught the importance of personal hygiene, such as clean underwear every day, and handwashing after visiting the lavatory. They should also know that too-frequent vaginal douches can wash away the protective mucous secretions.

The urinary tract is protected by a mucous lining, and the urine produced in the kidneys flushes out potentially harmful organisms. The pH reaction of the urine also prevents the multiplication of some organisms.

Some secretions, like tears, contain an enzyme *lysozyme* which helps to kill certain micro-organisms. Other secretions like the wax in the ears, and mucus from the respiratory tract, act as a defence because they are sticky, and dust containing micro-organisms adheres, and is then excreted. The respiratory tract is lined by special cells which produce hair-like projections called cilia, and other cells (goblet) produce mucus. Any dust containing micro-organisms which is inhaled, sticks to the mucus and is wafted up the tract from the lungs to be coughed out as sputum.

Prolonged heavy smoking not only causes the goblet cells to enlarge and secrete more mucus, but wears away the cilia so that the protective mechanism is lost.

Hairs which grow from the skin lining the lower part of the nose, and the external opening of the ears, act as a mechanical barrier.

The eyes are protected by the eyelids and lashes. The blink reflex protects against damage by bright light, and foreign particles, which are also washed away by tears.

There are many sites in, and on, the body where micro-organisms grow and multiply normally *(commensals)*. This is called the normal flora of the body, and helps in the protection by the 'crowding out' of potentially pathogenic organisms. This process can be likened to a person trying to get on a crowded underground train during the rush hour.

The intact skin acts as an effective barrier to infection in this way, as does the large intestine where organisms like the *E.coli* normally flourish, helping to break down food, and also helping to build up substances like certain vitamins which are needed by the body cells.

Mucous membranes protect the eyes, and line all parts of the body which have external openings, and when intact, help in the protection against invading organisms. The membranes are also highly vascular, which means that more blood carrying *phagocytes* (white cells which engulf foreign protein) can be brought to the area should a break in the continuity of the membrane allow pathogenic organisms to enter.

Inside the body, special lymphoid tissue acts as a filter by producing these white cells (phagocytes) which engulf foreign protein, like pathogenic micro-organisms. The tonsils are examples of this tissue, which can become enlarged and painful when active. Other tissues in the body, for example, bone marrow, and the spleen, produce *antibodies* which combine with foreign proteins, rendering them harmless so that the phagocytes can engulf and destroy them.

Causes of disease

(a) Genetic

Some diseases are genetic in origin — they are linked to the genes and are sometimes called hereditary. Haemophilia is a disease linked to the X chromosomes in the cell. It is transmitted from one generation to another — the symptoms being predominantly in the male.

(b) Congenital

Sometimes the individual is born with a condition which is apparent at birth or becomes so later, e.g. congenital dislocation of the hips, a cleft lip, or a heart imperfectly formed.

(c) Inflammatory

Inflammation is the response of body cells and tissues to injury occurring in any part of the body. The simplest example is the effect of friction on the skin, e.g. an ill-fitting shoe rubbing on the heel which is painful, becomes red, hot and

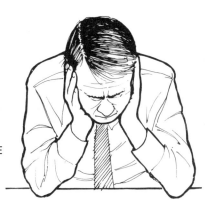

MENTAL DISORDERS

TRAUMATIC
(including radiation)

NEOPLASTIC

DEGENERATIVE

METABOLIC–ENDOCRINE
CHEMICAL POISONING

GENETIC

CONGENITAL

INFLAMMATORY
INFESTATION
INFECTIVE

AUTO–IMMUNE
ALLERGIC
PSYCHOSOMATIC
IATROGENIC

UNKNOWN ORIGIN

Figure 3.1   The causes of disease and disability

may become swollen, blistered and causes a limp. Some poisons irritate the kidney causing it to cease to function correctly because of inflammation, and concussion may cause inflammation of the brain tissue.

(d) Infective

Infectious diseases, such as mumps, whooping cough and measles, and also infections such as a boil, or a septic finger, are examples of disease due to infection — the successful invasion of the body tissues by pathogenic micro-organisms. Measures can be taken to prevent such illness or to lessen the severity of an attack of the disease. Immunisation of young babies is one method of reducing the likelihood and severity of measles or whooping cough, and the use of vaccine against poliomyelitis or influenza is another.

(e) Infestation

Disease may be caused by parasites — living organisms living at the expense of the human host. Examples include scabies, the itch mite burrowing into the skin, threadworms infesting the gut, and pediculosis — lice on the head, on the body or in the pubic and axillary hair.

(f) Traumatic

Trauma or injury is the cause of much misery and suffering. Accidents in the home, especially burns and scalds, account for a high proportion of accidents in Britain. Road and traffic accidents, major disasters in plane crashes or mining accidents are obvious causes of disability. The Royal Society for the Prevention of Accidents, the Health and Safety at Work Act and the legislation regarding the use and storage of poisonous substances are examples of the way in which attempts are made to control dangerous practices which might cause accidents.

Surgical treatment and dental extraction are examples of trauma caused intentionally to treat disease. Sunburn due to careless overexposure of the skin to ultraviolet light can cause severe burns, and the destruction of skin in extreme cases.

(g) Degenerative

Body cells and tissues degenerate and are replaced during infancy and child-hood very rapidly. In the adult, and with increasing age, the process of repair and renewal is less rapid and may fail completely. These processes of degeneration occur for example in bone and joints, in the ligaments binding bones together, in the blood vessels, and in the lens of the eye. The onset of such disease can be insidious, beginning in early middle age and showing its effects later according to the particular individual. These disease processes are not confined to the old and the elderly.

(h) Neoplastic

Neoplasm or new growth, is a term which covers *any* abnormal growth in the body. Benign tumours, i.e. those swellings or growths which are not due to cancer, can cause no symptoms, or they may be painful, cause abnormal irritation, or interference with the functions of the body, e.g. a cyst in the breast (a simple cyst is a space-filling capsule with fluid inside it).

Definitions

Carcinoma: Cancer arising from epithelial tissue, e.g. skin, gut, bladder, breast, air passages.
Sarcoma: Cancer arising from the connective and skeletal tissue (muscle, bone, cartilage).
Teratoma: Cancer arising from ovaries and testes.
Glioma: Cancer arising from nervous tissue.
Oncology: The study of neoplastic tumours.

Malignant disease is neoplasm — new growth — caused by abnormal cells which divide and subdivide, forming tumours, or breaking off and being carried in the lymphatic system and the blood circulation to form growths elsewhere. The first site for this cancerous growth, the primary site, may be treated by radiation or medication or may be excised (removed by surgery), but the spread of the disease in the body may already have occurred, causing secondary growths elsewhere.

(i) Metabolic

Diseases of metabolism include those of hormone or enzyme deficiency, e.g. phenylketonuria due to the deficiency of the enzyme alanine, or excessive activity or overproduction of hormones or enzymes. Examples of overactivity include the effect of imbalance of the growth hormone in the pituitary gland, causing abnormal height (gigantism), and the overproduction of hormone from the thyroid gland causing increased rate of metabolism (hyperthyroidism). Examples of deficiency include the failure to produce sufficient growth hormone in the pituitary gland causing dwarfism, and the failure of the pancreas to produce sufficient insulin, causing the disease called diabetes mellitus.

Chemical poisoning is sometimes classified under the heading of metabolic diseases — because poisons such as alcohol, drugs and poisonous plants affect the liver as well as having widespread effects on the body and its metabolism. Overeating, failure to eat and failure to absorb nutrients in infancy, are examples of nutritional disorders affecting the metabolism.

(j) Allergic

Hay fever and nettle rash are two common examples of allergy — a reaction by the body to a foreign protein substance. The condition is called an allergic response, and the cause of the problem is the allergen. Certain susceptible individuals respond to this foreign substance by an over-reaction producing a defensive mechanism far in excess of need. Some, in fact, are allergic to the protein in cow's milk or the foreign protein may be pollen grains in the air, or food, e.g. shellfish, strawberries, or from animals, birds, or other substances.

(k) Auto-immune response

In some individuals the body reacts by making attacks on its own tissues. The normal response to an injury in the tissues is an inflammation — the blood supply to the attacked tissue is increased, redness occurs — the white cells in the blood are active to overcome the invasion or irritation of the tissues, so there is local heat and swelling which may cause pain. In the normal response inflammation is a defence against injury. The cells make antibodies which attack invading bodies. In auto-immune disease the body over-reacts without any known cause and produces antibodies which affect its own tissues, e.g. rheumatoid arthritis, a disease affecting the joints, and other conditions affecting the thymus, and the thyroid gland.

(l) Psychosomatic

Some diseases are caused by a strong link between the mind and the body — the one affecting disease processes in the other. Since the human being is a unified whole, and mind and body interact throughout life, it could be argued that all diseases affect both the mind and body, but there are also certain known physical diseases affecting the body where the causes originate in the mind — the *psyche*. Examples include anxiety and stress which may induce or exacerbate ulcers in the duodenum or small intestine, and certain skin diseases.

(m) Mental disorders

Mental disorders are described in similar ways to diseases of the body by the effects they produce on the individual and the behaviour he shows as a result of the illness. Psychiatrists and psychiatric nurses are concerned with treating the individual and helping him and his family, or workmates, to achieve an understanding of his condition, and to cope with the challenges that daily living makes on his behaviour. There is a tendency to resist labelling and categorising the diseases, with the recognition that it is in living his life and coping with the environment, that help can best be given to the individual.

Mental illness such as depression can cause physical symptoms, and change in lifestyle, and the nurse needs to help the patient to fulfil the activities of daily living in order to maintain the health of his body.

(n) Iatrogenic

Iatrogenic illness as defined in *Dorland's Illustrated Medical Dictionary* (1974): *Iatro* (Greek) — physician and *Gennan* (Greek) — to produce. The term is now applied to any adverse condition in a patient occurring as the result of treatment by a physician or surgeon.

It is known that in certain serious illnesses one particular drug is effective in arresting the disease. Unfortunately the drug may produce side effects which cause distress to the patient, and which also have to be treated.

In prescribing such a drug, for example *cortisone,* sometimes used in the treatment of chronic bronchial asthma, the doctor uses his professional judgement based on a sound knowledge of the evidence, and after carefully weighing up all the pros and cons of the situation.

In some patients, drugs such as *antibiotics,* given to counteract infecting organisms, can alter the normal flora of the body, allowing other and sometimes more dangerous organisms to invade and multiply.

Illich (1981) states that 'the medical establishment has become a major threat to health' and while not everyone would necessarily agree with that statement, it is true that certain treatments prescribed by the doctor can produce adverse effects in the patient.

(o) Unknown origin

Medical science continues to advance, but aetiology — the study of the causation of disease — is still incomplete, and some diseases are of unknown origin. In such instances, the description of the condition enables diagnosis to be made, treatment or relief to be offered, and even the prognosis of the disease to be indicated, without its exact cause being yet known.

Definitions

Diagnosis: the nature of the disease inferred by symptoms and signs.
Prognosis: the forecast course of a disease and its outcome.

Infection

Infection may be defined as 'the successful invasion of the body by pathogenic micro-organisms'.

Pathogens are capable of producing disease and may be broadly divided into three groups: bacteria, fungi, and viruses. The human body can live in health and yet carry disease-producing organisms — the body is, therefore, sometimes referred to as a reservoir of pathogens. While these organisms cause no harm to the individual they are called 'commensals', but if they gain entry to other sites in the body, or to another person's body, they may then produce disease i.e. infection. Wherever people meet, make contact by shaking hands, kissing, or close contact or when people live together in a confined space it is possible for organisms to be carried from one person to another. This is particularly likely to cause infection if these people are already ill with other diseases, or if they are not receiving proper nutrition, or if there is inadequate ventilation. Colds spread rapidly from one student to another in overheated rooms with no windows opened!

(a) Pathogenic organisms

The requirements for growth of these single-celled organisms are similar to those of the human body. The normal warmth of the human body encourages them to reproduce, and it has been calculated that one single bacterium can reproduce to form 262 144 bacteria within 6 hours, as each subdivides!

The invasion of the body tissues may be:

- By inhalation during breathing, from droplets in the air, or dust.
- By inoculation through the skin from an insect bite, thorn or pin.
- By absorption from the intestinal tract in water or digested food material.
- By direct contact — skin or mucous membrane, on the feet, or in kissing, or sexual intercourse, on the eyelids and conjunctiva.
- By blood from mother to baby across the placenta in utero.

When a person is ill, the body is already at risk, with the metabolic processes called upon to maintain or restore health; the ability to resist the invasion of organisms is therefore greatly reduced. Once the pathogens have invaded the tissues (e.g. left the intestinal tract and are absorbed or have crossed from the air into the alveoli and then to the blood) they may multiply, and cause the person to be the *host.* The host for these disease-producing organisms is a potential source of danger to other people:

1. Whilst he is incubating the infection (i.e. before the signs of a successful invasion appear).
2. Whilst he is suffering the symptoms of infection.

3. Whilst he is convalescing from the infection.
4. Whilst he is suffering from a sub-clinical infection, i.e. one that goes no further than stage (1) and he does not know he is infected.

Definition

Sub-clinical: infection present but not showing the clinical symptoms or 5: When he has become a permanent carrier of the organism without symptoms.

(b) The potential victim

The victim is at risk if his health is already affected by disease, or if his powers of resistance are lowered by age, infirmity or frailty. The very old and the very young have less resistance, and may succumb to gastrointestinal infection, or to influenza or colds. Outbreaks of food poisoning or influenza may cause deaths in residential homes, or in hospitals for the elderly or for children.

(c) Response to infection in the body

1 Cellular response

Firstly, the cells in the body at the site of infection respond and cells from the blood, the white cells — leucocytes — attack the invading organisms. This response results in local inflammation, and the outcome may be successful, so that the organisms are destroyed; possibly also some cells die, but the white cells remove the destroyed matter by a process called ingestion — they render harmless the debris by taking it into themselves. This activity of white cells is called phagocytosis.

2 Antibody response

Some pathogens stimulate the body to form antibodies, specific substances which counteract the effects they produce. The pathogen is the antigen which stimulates the body to produce an antibody in response to this attack. This stimulus may be sufficient to enable the person to develop actively an immunity to further attacks by similar pathogens, and to protect the individual when exposed again to similar organisms.

3 Toxins and antitoxins

Some pathogens, when they have invaded the body tissues, produce a harmful substance called toxin, which enters the bloodstream and is carried to one of the organs of the body where it causes damage. The toxin from the pathogen causing diphtheria may travel in the blood and cause paralysis by damaging the nervous system, although the organism which is the cause of the toxin does not enter the bloodstream.

Antitoxins may also be produced by the human body to counteract specific toxins, and to overcome their effects. The person who has the disease, or is convalescing from the disease may have a plentiful supply of antitoxins in the blood.

Antitoxin, specially prepared under laboratory conditions, may be prescribed in the treatment of diphtheria. The patient is given the antitoxin as a form of passive immunity to prevent further damage by the diphtheria toxin.

N.B. Toxoid is a preparation of treated toxin, attenuated, i.e. made less harmful, which may be injected in a small amount, and repeated at scheduled intervals to stimulate the healthy body to produce its own antitoxin without suffering from the disease. This is to encourage active immunity, and is the rationale for the immunisation of infants and young children, e.g. triple vaccine is diphtheria toxoid, whooping cough vaccine and tetanus toxoid. Three injections are needed at intervals with booster doses later, to maintain the immunity, at pre-school and school age.

Pathogenic bacteria which overcome the local response may gain entry to the bloodstream, causing bacteraemia, or the toxins they produce may circulate and cause toxaemia, or organisms and the debris and infected material may circulate in the bloodstream causing septicaemia.

Viruses are very small single-celled organisms which penetrate the cell membrane of surface cells in the body surfaces, e.g. in the orifices and cavities of the respiratory tract, the intestinal tract, the vulva and vagina, and spread from cell to cell. When viruses enter the bloodstream they cause viraemia, a

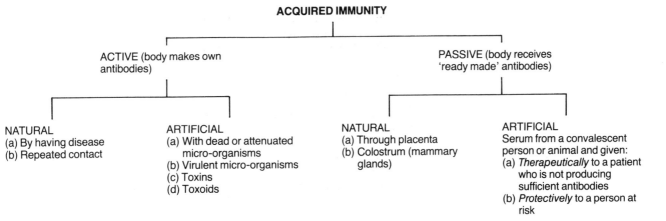

ACQUIRED IMMUNITY

ACTIVE (body makes own antibodies)

NATURAL
(a) By having disease
(b) Repeated contact

ARTIFICIAL
(a) With dead or attenuated micro-organisms
(b) Virulent micro-organisms
(c) Toxins
(d) Toxoids

PASSIVE (body receives 'ready made' antibodies)

NATURAL
(a) Through placenta
(b) Colostrum (mammary glands)

ARTIFICIAL
Serum from a convalescent person or animal and given:
(a) *Therapeutically* to a patient who is not producing sufficient antibodies
(b) *Protectively* to a person at risk

Figure 3.2   Classification of immunity

very serious condition. The virus will only grow and reproduce within a living cell — it is therefore very difficult to treat as any substance used to destroy it would damage the body cells. It also cannot live except in living cells, and can therefore only be grown in the laboratory in living tissue, such as a developing hen's egg, or tissue cultures from mice or rat's tissue.

The body's immune system is discussed further in chapter 8 of Hunt and Sendell's *Nursing the Adult with a Specific Physiological Disturbance*.

(d) The spread of infection

Environmental spread of pathogens from the host to potential victim may be:

Airborne — on droplets from breathing, coughing and sneezing.
— from droplets falling to the floor, and raised in dust, particularly those organisms which form spores to resist adverse conditions.

Waterborne — by contaminated water supplies.
— from sewage to water and food supplies.
— by water already contaminated used in preparing food.

Food — in milk — tuberculous cow or adulterated milk supply.
— in eggs — particularly duck eggs — too lightly cooked.
— in processed meat pies and other products, or frozen chickens.
— by warming up 'previously cooked foods'.
— in ice cream and custard and cream cakes.

Insect — by mosquito bites.
— by flies or other insects contaminating uncovered food.

Animals — by mice, rats, cats and dogs.

Lack of hygiene, particularly in food handling, and failure to wash the hands after defaecation and before preparing food, are the most frequent causes of outbreaks of diarrhoea and vomiting in children, in the elderly and in the communities living in hostels, camps and other such accommodation.

Food poisoning

Definition

Acute inflammation of the gastrointestinal tract after eating food containing harmful matter.

(a) Causes of food poisoning

1. Vegetable poisons — plants, berries, fungi.
2. Chemical poisons — lead, zinc, arsenic.

Commonest cause

3. Pathogenic micro-organisms in food.

1 Salmonella group of bacteria

1. From carrier with bacteria in the gastrointestinal tract, and then by meat, milk and dairy produce handled by carrier.
2. From meat infected by bacteria.
3. From milk from infected animals.
4. From eggs — duck eggs especially (need to be boiled for 14 min to kill salmonella).
5. Flies from faeces to food.
6. Rats and mice as above, or as disease carriers.

Salmonella are living organisms needing warmth and moisture to grow and reproduce — they are destroyed by high temperature, i.e. in baking or boiling. Keeping food warm or heating up increases their rate of reproduction, e.g. in soup, or custard or casseroles. Insufficient cooking of frozen chicken, or failure to defrost poultry before cooking, is a common cause.

2 Staphylococci

Certain strains produce a poisonous substance — a toxin — as they grow and reproduce which is particularly harmful to the gastrointestinal tract — and it is therefore called an enterotoxin.

Staphylococci may be carried to food during preparation or in the sale and distribution, or when serving meals:

1. From boils, or septic fingers, or infected spots.
2. From the air breathed out when bacteria in droplets of water fall on to the food, or by sneezing, coughing and careless use of disposable tissues by those with a respiratory infection, such as a cold or cough.

The enterotoxin is not always destroyed by cooking, which kills staphylococci. N.B.: Healthy people do carry these organisms on the hands and in the nostrils, and therefore scrupulous hand washing is essential before touching food to prevent contamination.

The prevention of cross-infection

In hospital wards, clinics and residential homes or schools the possibility of spreading infection from host to victim is clearly increased. In hospital wards, in spite of all attempts to the contrary, the level of organisms in air, on food and on equipment is very high. Such organisms have also adapted to their environment, and they have developed strains which are able to resist the attempts to destroy them, i.e. antibiotic-resistant strains have developed. Antibiotics are a form of medication developed to act against bacterial pathogens without harming living cells — penicillin is a well-known example.

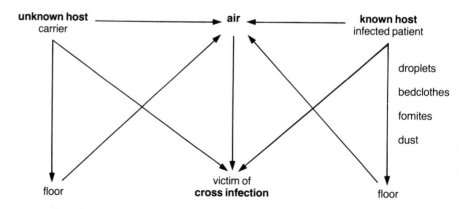

Figure 3.3   Possible ways of spreading infection from one person to another in wards and in the home

Nursing staff can help to prevent infection spreading from one patient to another, or from staff to patients, however, by applying knowledge of microbiology, by practising high standards of personal cleanliness, and by encouraging others to do likewise.

(a) Hands

Research has shown the areas of her own body which the nurse's hands touch during a span of duty, Taylor (1978) has also demonstrated how ineffective hand washing can be by nursing staff. Since the nurse's hands are the tools of her trade, effective care of the nails and skin of the hands as well as careful washing and drying between each activity she carries out, is an important aspect in preventing the nurse causing harm to her patient. Nails need to be kept short, with massage to the cuticle. The use of a suitable barrier cream or hand cream nightly will be helpful to prevent dryness of the skin — a cause in itself of possible infection. Patients should be taught and encouraged to wash the hands carefully after visiting the lavatory for micturition or defaecation; and after the patient has used the commode, or bedpan or urinal, the nurse should provide the means of hand washing.

Microbiologists have demonstrated the 'finger faecal' cycle which shows how failure to wash the hands afer defaecation, or after emptying bedpans, or changing a baby's napkin, can carry pathogenic micro-organisms to the patients' food, the baby's bottle or to the nurse herself at her next meal. Outbreaks of severe diarrhoea and vomiting can be traced from one patient to another — spread by nursing staff in this way. This is possible particularly in wards or homes caring for the very young or very frail elderly persons.

(b) Ventilation

Adequate ventilation of the room where the patient is being nursed, or of the ward, is very important to prevent the spread of organisms from the air; coughing and sneezing projects bacteria and viruses into the air over a wide range.

In treatment rooms surgical dressings should be removed from wounds with as little contact as possible, with the contaminated side of the dressing being exposed to the air for the briefest time before it is disposed of in a paper bag to be incinerated.

Although cold draughts should be avoided, the opening of windows for fresh air to circulate not only helps to prevent the contamination of the air but it also stimulates and refreshes the patient who cannot leave his bed.

(c) Household cleanliness

The nurse is responsible for the patient's environment — to safeguard him from harm. Therefore, although the ward sister or charge nurse is not in charge of the domestic arrangements, and the nursing staff are not required to clean the wards, she is nevertheless the person who sets the standard of cleanliness expected from the household staff. The ward sister and the household supervisor should maintain close links to enable the patients' setting to be clean and regularly cleaned. Dust from the air and the movement of bedclothes and equipment settles on furniture, particularly on the patients' lockers or bedtables. It falls on the floor, and organisms from the roads, soil and surroundings are carried on footwear, and settle in the dust, together with the organisms that fall in the droplets as patients and staff breathe out, cough or sneeze. Some of these organisms form spores which remain in the dust and withstand adverse conditions. Vacuum or suction cleaning and dusting with mop or duster impregnated with an anti-static material daily or twice daily is therefore usual. The patient's fruit bowl, or tray with water or fruit squash, needs washing regularly, and as little equipment as possible should be left at the bedside.

(d) Sinks and baths

The use of communal sinks, baths or washing bowls is a potential hazard to the safety of the patient. After bathing, or washing, the patient should be encouraged to rinse the bath or sink — helped by the nurse if necessary. When preparing for the patient to have a bath in the bathroom, the nurse should make sure the bath is clean, using the preparation supplied for this, and rinsed before running the bath water and collecting her patient.

Household detergents, supplied in well-labelled containers, should not be left where children or confused patients may use them for other purposes. It is particularly important that no bleach or other chemically poisonous solutions should be left in the bathroom. The safety of staff and patients requires that no household cleaning lotions should be emptied into fruit juice bottles, or any other receptacle associated with food or drink.

Bath mats (like swimming baths and baths) may harbour pathogenic micro-organisms, particularly the fungus which causes 'athlete's foot'. The patient should be helped to step on to his own bath mat or a disposable mat, or on to his own slipper, to prevent contamination. Washing bowls for patients washing or being washed in bed should be washed and rinsed after use, before being returned for use again by another patient. On no account should the same bowl be used for several patients, not only would this be socially unacceptable, it is also a harmful practice, as a source of cross-infection.

(e) Lavatories, commodes and bedpans

These should be cleaned at least once in 24 hours, by domestic staff, using a proprietary cleanser, hot water, clean cloths and elbow grease! The nursing staff should then make sure that each is carefully emptied, cleaned and rinsed after use by each patient. Most wards have special equipment for emptying and sterilising bedpans after each time of use! A disinfectant liquid is usually provided for any mops or forceps used for handling faecally-contaminated material.

Definitions

Sterilise: to remove all living organisms.
Disinfect: to attempt to destroy harmful pathogens.
Disinfectant: a chemical solution which will destroy pathogenic bacteria in a suitable time, and strength.

N.B. Care should be taken to keep such lotions away from patient areas, and away from children in the home.

Most disinfectants will be harmful to the skin, or if splashed into the eye — first aid includes rinsing with cold water at once if this occurs.

Activity

1. List the disinfectants in use in your training school giving:
   (a) The purpose for which they are used.
   (b) The strength of the lotion.
   (c) The time needed for them to be useful.
2. What other means of disinfection are there?
3. Some health districts have a nurse who is a 'Control of infection nursing officer'.
   What would such a nurse do?
   How would she carry out her work?

Some hospitals have disposable bedpans. In others the nurse has to empty the contents of the bedpan down the sluice hopper, rinse the bedpan with cold water, then check it is empty before washing and drying. Sometimes a commode or bedpan is kept for one patient who has a particular infection, and if this is so it should be carefully marked and kept in a special place, not returned for use in the general stock. Using a bedpan or commode in a public ward can be very embarrassing to a patient, even if his bed is curtained from view. The smell can embarrass also and the nursing student should use tact and understanding in the use of deodorisers and in ventilation.

(f) Bedclothes and patients' clothes

Each patient should have a place on his locker for his own face flannel and towel, bath towel and bath flannel, bedroom slippers and dressing gown. The bedclothes from his bed — counterpane, blankets, sheets and pillows should not be placed on other patients' beds. In bed making, as little disturbance should be created as possible to prevent raising and circulating the dust with its potential spores from the floor.

(g) Ward kitchen and food preparation

The cleanliness of the kitchen and the preparation of meals will also be undertaken by the domestic or household staff. The nurse may, however, be required to prepare milk drinks or to prepare fruit for her patient. She should begin by washing and drying her hands, collecting equipment first, then the milk, fruit or other food, and preparing it to take to her patient on a tray.

Cooperation between nursing and household staff, both of whom are working for the benefit of the patients, is essential, and a mutual understanding of each other's role can be developed by care and courtesy in order to maintain a neat clean environment within the ward.

The patients' problems — identified — assisted — the outcome considered

'There is a growing awareness that knowledge from many different fields must be used by nurses in identifying, defining and finding solutions to complex health care problems which individual nurses and patients are expected to solve within a a system of daily living which relates nurses to patients and to others who assist patients' (Orem, 1981).

Biological, social, psychological and medical sciences contribute to the understanding of human needs. Aspects of these sciences are helpful to the nursing student as she learns how to plan and give care to her patient. Pharmacology, nutrition and microbiology will contribute to her understanding of the needs of her patient, and to the treatment he is receiving and will anticipate the possible progress of his illness, the side effects of his treatment, and the change in his environment which may become necessary. Her nursing studies should be based on the understanding of health — health needs and health education — and on the prevention of disease in order that her care of the person who is ill will be planned realistically to reflect his lifestyle and his future needs within his family or work environment.

At the beginning of her course of training the nursing student also needs to learn something of the causes of illness in order to understand the effects it may have on the patient, and the modifications which will have to be made to his daily activities as a consequence.

The changes caused by disease are observed by the patient, or the nurse and the doctor. These are called the signs of the condition or disease. The patient may complain of pain, being breathless, tired or unable to move, and these are called symptoms. Relief of symptoms requires knowledge, forethought and planning. The nurse will record her observations, so that an estimate of the effects of treatment can be made.

(a) Sleep

A patient who cannot sleep should be given a warm drink, an opportunity to pass urine, and be made comfortable in bed — and be able to talk to a sympathetic nurse if he wishes, before a sedative is given. The actual hours of sleep or dozes should be noted, and if he is in pain, which prevents sleep, this should be reported at once.

(b) Rest

Rest is a means of treatment for many diseases, and a patient may often need encouragement to rest — particularly if he feels able to do more than his treatment indicates.

(c) Immobility

Some patients are unable to move at home or in hospital because of their disease, others have to remain in bed as part of their treatment. For whatever reason this occurs, lack of movement can be a hazard. In health, the human body is constantly moving, although this may not be obvious. Very few people sit absolutely still, for example, an artist's model or a keen birdwatcher have to learn how to control small movements — too small to catch the eye of a 'normal' observer. Locomotion, or moving from place to place, provides stimulation, and relief from boredom.

(d) Walking

This exercises muscles, keeping them (and the leg muscles in particular) in a state of 'tone'. The contraction of the muscles, i.e. moving the limbs at the joints, also causes pressure on the veins which are deep in the muscles of the leg so that the blood in the veins is moved upwards towards the heart. Inactive leg muscles cause potential stagnation of blood in the veins which can lead to disease and possible death of the patient. Walking and other exercises also affect breathing and stimulate the blood circulation and the intake of oxygen in the lungs.

(e) Exercise in bed

Even if the patient cannot walk or get up, he can be taught and encouraged to contract and relax his calf muscles, to breathe deeply and to exercise his arms if possible.

(f) Alteration of habit

The person who has to come into hospital for whatever cause, has to face a restriction on the amount of movement he can make — this is seen at its extreme if he has to rest completely in bed because of his condition and he is unable to wash or feed himself. Such rest may be life-saving, e.g. after a 'heart attack' — 'myocardial infarction' — but it also can give rise to problems caused by lack of movement. Noticeably, lack of movement interferes with bowel function causing constipation. Healthy individuals vary in the amount and timing of bowel actions, but each has an habitual action which is easily upset by changes in diet and lack of exercise.

(g) Pressure on the skin

Lack of movement means that the patient's weight will rest on the dependent part of the body, compressing the skin against the underlying subcutaneous tissue and bone. If the blood supply to the tissues in the surrounding area is reduced, or cut off, the tissue cells will begin to die and a purplish red area of skin may be seen, from which an ulcer will develop unless active treatment is undertaken quickly. This is a real hazard of immobility and the hazard of skin breakdown is increased under other conditions — when there is existing debilitating disease, lack of nutrition, loss of consciousness or sensation. Fever, and in the elderly with degenerative changes, urinary incontinence, lack of care in bedmaking, and failure to move the patient at least every 2 hours are possible causes of pressure sores which could have been prevented by nursing attention based on observation, sound knowledge of physiology and the research findings of Norton *et al.* (1975).

(h) Impaired balance causing potential injury

Sometimes the patient can move in a limited way, and his postural balance may be affected by this, e.g. he has to learn how to walk in a different way, after 'a stroke' (a cerebral vascular accident). Sometimes disorders of postural balance cause momentary dizziness — the patient feels giddy, and may fall down. In disease affecting some parts of the brain, the patient may have a seizure or fit in which he falls to the ground.

(i) Impaired vision

Partial loss of sight may cause the patient to stumble or not to be able to see at the edges of a range of vision. The nurse is therefore responsible for anticipating difficulties and hazards in the patient's path — moving his locker on to the side unaffected by paralysis or limited vision, and remaining within call and in the bathroom with the patient who may be attacked by faintness or a seizure.

Activity

BLINDFOLD

Ask a friend to blindfold you completely and to take you for a short walk out of doors, crossing roads and then indoors going up and down stairs. After this, ask her to feed you with a meal.
What have you learned:
1. About yourself?
2. About the limitations of blindness?
3. About your friend?

(j) Encouraging independence

Every adult values his own independence, to a greater or lesser degree. Some patients who are ill at home or come into hospital feel very acutely their loss of independence. Decisions are made on behalf of all patients about routine in the ward, e.g. mealtimes are set, medical staff consultations are forecast, and there are rules regarding the use of television or radios which are made for the common good, but which are new experiences for the particular patients. Some hospitals also have rules regarding visiting times and the arrangements for the use of outgoing telephone calls varies. Most hospitals provide a booklet about the facilities available for patients, and their visitors, with useful information about personal laundry, telephone numbers, chaplaincy services, hospital trolley shop and so on. The nursing student at the outset of the course will do well to pause and consider the very different environment that a hospital ward offers to the new patient. In many instances the ward is a bedroom, bathroom, lavatory, dining room and visitors' room for the patient, and his fellow patients. It is a place well known and taken for granted by nursing and medical and other paramedical and ancillary staff, but which is unknown and foreign to him. It may be the first time that he has experienced living in a community or social group. The nursing staff will be relied upon by this patient to help him to unravel the mysteries around him. Above all else, the nurse is the person who will maintain his sense of personal worth and self-esteem. No matter what his illness or his treatment she must see that he does not suffer from a loss of dignity as a human being. The person must come to no harm in her care. Respect for his person, his privacy, his name, and his belongings rests with the nurse.

References

Dorland's Illustrated Medical Dictionary, 25th edn, Saunders, Philadelphia, 1974

Hunt, J., The Teaching and Practice of Surgical Dressings in Three Hospitals, RCN, 1974

Illich, I., Limits to Medicine: Medical Nemesis, The Expropriation of Health, Penguin Books, p. 11, 1981

Nightingale, F., Notes on Nursing — What it is and What it is Not, Harrison and Sons London, 1st edn, 1859. See also Nightingale, F. and Skeet, M., Notes on Nursing, Churchill Livingstone, Edinburgh, 1980

Norton, D., McClaren, R. and Exton Smith, A., An Investigation of Geriatric Nursing Problems in Hospital, Churchill Livingstone, 1975

Orem, D. E., Nursing: Concepts of Practice, McGraw-Hill, 1981

Taylor, L. J., An evaluation of handwashing techniques, Nursing Times, No. 74, 1978

Volicer, B.J. and Bohammon, M.W., A hospital stress rating scale, Nursing Research, 2, 358, 1975

Further reading

Bergnam, R., Evaluation of nursing care — could it make a difference?, International Journal of Nursing Studies, 19 (2), 1982

Cartwright, A., Human Relations and Hospital Care, Routledge and Keegan Paul, 1974

Cox, C., Frontiers of nursing in the 21st century, International Journal of Nursing Studies, 19 (1), 1982

Franklin, B., Patient Anxiety on Admission to Hospital, RCN, 1974

Howarth, H., Mouth care procedures for the very ill, Nursing Times, 1977

Hunt, J., Nursing Care Plans. The Nursing Process at Work, Education for Care, H.M. and M., and Marks-Maran, D., 1980

McGhee, A., The Patient's Attitude to Nursing Care, Churchill Livingstone, 1961

Skeet, M., Home From Hospital, Dan Mason Research Publications, 1970

Chapter 4   Care of the dying and the bereaved

Emotional aspects *(by Barbara J. McNulty)*

Though death is the common end of all of us, it is the eventuality for which we make the least preparation. It is equally true that though every patient who comes under our care will ultimately die (in the present illness or at some other time) the possibility plays little or no part in our planning of his care. We confidently assume that he will of course get better, and all our efforts are directed towards that end. For 90% of the patients in a general ward our attitude will be appropriate, but for the remaining 10% with whom we are at present concerned, our assumptions are totally inappropriate, and our care will necessarily be so also.

The first requirement in caring for the dying patient is the recognition of the true state of affairs. He is dying. This is not a defeatist attitude but one based on reality; one which will ensure that the treatment and care given are appropriate to the patient's needs. His needs will be emotional as well as physical and they will change with the course of his illness, often from day to day or even hour to hour. The nurse must be alert to these signs of change and adjust her care accordingly.

In the early days the patient will probably be denying the evident gravity of his illness. He will be looking on the bright side, hoping for a cure, making plans for the future. He will be wanting confirmation of his hopes from those about him and will not be ready to have them denied. At this stage it is appropriate to go along with him in his hopes, but with cautious optimism only. No unrealistic promises should be made, or rash assurances given. As the illness progresses he will begin to have doubts and fears that perhaps all is not so well and these doubts may manifest themselves in outbursts of anger and frustration. The target for this anger may be 'they' or it may be God, or it may be directed at the hospital, a doctor or a nurse, or it may be the wife or daughter who is bitterly attacked. These are hard days, for mostly the anger is quite irrational and the blame quite undeserved. There is no reasoning with him and little comfort for his victim. Families need much reassurance that this phase will pass and that it is not really they with whom he is so angry. The important factor here is to keep the lines of communication open, keep oneself in contact with the patient, reassure him that no matter what he says or does, one believes in him and cares about him and will not run away.

As this phase burns itself out and the patient continues to deteriorate, there is often a withdrawal into himself. In direct contrast to his outbursts of anger he is now silent, brooding, withdrawn and isolated in his grief for what is happening to him. Our words will not reach him in this next phase only expert physical care with infinite attention to detail and careful observation of symptoms will ensure that some bond of communication is maintained between him and his attendants. Until at last the first tentative questions will begin to come, and one must recognise the change in what is being asked. Previously the optimistically phrased 'I know it will take a long time' only required agreement. But now the more direct 'It doesn't look so good does it?' requires either an opening up of the discussion by 'I wonder what makes you say that?' or an endorsement of what he has said by saying something like 'Well, no, it's not as good as we had hoped'. One's knowledge of the patient and one's appreciation of the subtle way in which his questions have changed will tell us that he is looking for confirmation of what he now already knows, i.e. that his illness is fatal. It is at this point that the nurse must be prepared to stand her ground. No lies will fool him now, he *knows,* and he needs someone who will share his knowing. No direct statement is required of us, only a willingness to listen and a quiet acceptance of what he is telling us. More than anything else he needs someone to whom he can voice his fears and anxieties without the danger of being 'cheered up'.

The whole aim of terminal care must be to relieve distress where ever possible; pain, nausea, sleeplessness, breathlessness, discomfort of every kind must be taken seriously, observed and monitored, hourly if necessary, and the drugs and nursing care adjusted accordingly. Whereas it may have been appropriate one week to sit a patient out in a chair for a while, the next week this may be quite beyond, not necessarily his physical ability, but his emotional needs. If he is just coming to the realisation that he is dying it may be a relief to him to know that he need not go on fighting but can lie down and rest. Patients try so hard to please, to do what is expected of them, it is important that we temper our expectations to their capacities, without too many set ideas of how it should or should not be. Often a serving of a hitherto forbidden but favourite dish may do more for him that the strict adherence to a diet. Or a totally contraindicated visit home, however exhausting, may be more beneficial to his spirit, than the prescribed bed rest could possible be for his body. One must be flexible in one's approach to what a dying person should or should not do, and he must be the arbiter of how his last days shall be lived.

The need to recognise the truth of the situation is not confined to the patient and his medical and nursing staff. The family also needs to know and will need help in understanding and coming to terms with their impending loss. They will need a clear statement of facts given gently, truthfully and in language they can understand. Hurried, embarrassed half truths given apologetically, will not do. The situation calls for time, privacy, sympathy, honesty and the ability to enter into another person's distress without being overwhelmed by it. To enable the family to make the best use of the time left to them they need help in learning to share with the patient their thoughts, fears and grief about the future. This sharing is hard to initiate, particularly if communication within the family has been poor for some time. Often both relative and patient have known the diagnosis, but each has refrained from speaking of it for fear of distressing the other. Yet once sharing has been achieved their mutual support of one another can be a source of strength and satisfaction to them both. One way of helping a couple to bridge the silent gap between them is by saying to each privately 'I think Mary/John is worrying about you, have you tried to talk to her/him? I think this would be helpful'. Often this little bit of encouragement is all that is needed.

Many a dying patient's intractable pain or persistent insomnia are heightened by his emotional state. No amount of analgesia or sedation will cure the pain of grief or silence the deep anxieties that haunt him. While correct medication and adequate analgesia are essential to his comfort, only the sharing of his grief and anxieties will bring him peace of mind. A direct question is often the best way of approaching the subject. 'You're looking tired/sad this morning Mr Jones. I expect you're worrying about yourself/your family a bit, can I help?' Sit down as you say it, make it clear that you have got time to talk, take his hand, show that you are concerned and want to help.

Our aim must always be to unite the family, to try and strengthen the bonds between them. If there is a 'black sheep' who has not been heard of for years, every effort should be made to trace him. If there is a family feud (and what family does not have them) now is the time to try and heal the wounds. The patient will die with one less pain on his conscience and the bereaved will be left with a sense of achievement and a strange satisfaction that all was well. It is the things left unsaid and the actions left undone which haunt the bereaved with a sense of guilt. 'If only I had told him', 'If only I had done what I meant to do', are phrases commonly heard. If only, if only, and now it is too late. The final weeks of an illness are important both for the patient and for the family. This will be the last spring, or the last birthday, or the last Sunday. It is part of our caring to make these 'last' times worth having and worth remembering.

The care of the dying and their families is one of the most rewarding aspects of nursing, but we so often spoil it for ourselves by being afraid of doing the wrong thing or of not being able to cope. Yet what is called for is quite simple — our expert nursing skills and a sensitive and caring attitude. The object of our care is a person undergoing the greatest experience of his life and we are privileged to share some part of the experience with him.

Care of the dying

The person whose life is drawing to a close should not be left alone. If friends or relatives are unable to be present then a nurse, or a student of nursing, should sit beside the bed, to comfort, to support and to care for the dying person.

It is a responsible service to care for such a patient, and it is not a frightening experience if the young nursing student is properly prepared for this privilege.

As life ebbs away slowly, the systems of the body cease to function. The physical senses and emotions may be heightened before this occurs, and therefore the nurse should keep her voice low, appear calm and caring, and comfort by her touch, e.g. by holding the patient's hand, smoothing the hair from the brow, and moistening the lips with a damp tissue.

Whenever consciousness is lost, e.g. under an anaesthetic, or as a result of illness, the sense of hearing persists when other senses are lost. The nurse treating an unconscious patient should remember this, and particularly when there are periods of sleeping, waking and lapsing into unconsciousness.

The dying person can take great comfort from a soft voice, reading from a prayer book, from a book of poetry, or reading letters to him. The nurse should observe the patient, to see if he has a Bible, a copy of the Koran, or any other reading material beside him. It is not easy to converse with someone who cannot reply verbally, but the pressure of the hand, a fleeting smile, or a change of expression will indicate if the contact is welcomed.

Relatives and friends

Relatives and friends can be helped to appreciate that their presence is helpful. Often they like to help with simple tasks — such as keeping the hair off the face, dampness on the forehead, a lip salve on the lips, or when swallowing is impossible, damp tissue or cotton wool to moisten the tongue. Visitors should, however, be watched carefully for any signs that they are becoming too distressed. A cup of tea, and an opportunity to sit quietly in a waiting room may help them, or the suggestion that they should go for a short walk in the fresh air. An understanding nurse will encourage them to talk, to weep, or to remain quiet, as they wish. The chaplain, or an appropriate minister of religion, will be available, and should be contacted, if needed. It is a comfort, at such times, if the patient can be seen to appear calm, resting at peace and in a clean and tidy room.

Religious aspects for particular groups

Romany families set great store by being with the family members at the time of death, and a large number of a 'tribe' will need to be given the use of a nearby waiting room.

Muslims expect to sit with a dying relative — a man with a man, if possible, so that they may sit, pray with and touch the patient. A woman will sit with her husband who is dying but will never touch him in any way.

Roman Catholics receive the Sacrament of the Sick (previously called the Last Rites or Extreme Unction) which consists of anointing the forehead and hands with holy oils. Communion may also be given at the same time if the patient is conscious and can swallow — sips of water should be given afterwards.

Signs of death

The patient may lose consciousness before there is any change in respiratory rate and depth, and before there are changes in heart beat and pulse rate.

Sometimes there are lapses between the conscious and unconscious state. When conscious, the weight of bedclothes or nightdress may distress the patient, and a dry mouth or lips can be very disturbing even after the swallowing reflex is lost and the patient is unable to swallow, or to absorb fluids given orally, or by a naso-oesophageal tube. Dentures may be removed if this makes the patient more comfortable. There are changes in the colour of the skin, which is more obvious in the face — the cheeks and nose, and ear lobes losing colour and becoming cold. The nails and fingers also change in colour, and there is very little change when slight pressure is put upon the nail bed. The skin on the trunk and extremities may become blotchy, as the blood circulation ceases. The respirations may become slow, with periods between each breath lengthening, and this is called apnoea. Sometimes the changes in the rate and depth of breathing are accompanied by noisy breathing caused by moist air passages, and in the absence of the cough reflex, this can be distressing to those caring for the patient, even though the patient is not distressed by it (in lay terms the 'death rattle'). This may be relieved if the doctor prescribes an injection to assist in lessening the secretion of mucus, which may be more comforting for the patient than the use of gentle suction by the nurse through a special catheter in the nasopharynx.

The person who is dying may have other symptoms requiring relief or treatment, and the appropriate care plan will indicate if this is so.

When the pulse becomes weak, and 'thready', and imperceptible, and the respirations cease, the nurse in charge should be notified, and the medical officer is sent for to certify that death has occurred. The patient should then be left in an appropriate position, so that relatives or friends can remain with him for a few moments alone before being taken to a quiet room for a cup of tea and a talk with the nurse in charge.

The care of the body

As soon as the relatives and friends have left, the body should be laid flat in bed, in the recumbent position (i.e. flat on the back) with no pillow. The dentures can be re-inserted, and any rings removed, according to the wishes of the patient's next of kin, or any left on covered with adhesive plaster.

The jaw should be pushed forward, and held by a soft pillow under the chin, or by a bandage, secured in place. The feet should be placed together, the nightwear removed, and the body left covered by a sheet.

It is usual to leave the body for an hour before washing. The body is then placed in a shroud, or clean nightwear, and wrapped in a sheet with labels on the body and the sheet, giving the name of the patient. Different hospitals have differing methods of carrying out the details of this procedure. It is therefore essential that you should become familiar with the method used in your own training school.

It is always essential to be sensitive and respectful, as well as competent, when treating the patient who has died. This is the last service offered by the nursing staff and will be remembered by the relatives and friends as an experience when nursing was really 'caring'.

Cultural and religious differences should also be observed after the patient has died.

Orthodox Jews do not allow any further treatment by the nursing staff. The Rabbi or a relative will arrange for 'a watcher' and special arrangements with an undertaker.

Muslims believe that the body should be burned as soon as possible after the death to prevent the soul suffering. In the home, where circumstances allow, there are special ceremonies and prayers by family and friends prior to an early cremation. In hospital when a Muslim patient dies, it is usual for the care of the body to be carried out, and then taken direct to the local Mosque where special ceremonies are arranged when home circumstances do not permit this to take place.

Death in the family* *(by Stephen Kirkham)*

The occurrence of a death in a family means that there is a testing time ahead for the bereaved. There will be emotional and practical difficulties. This article will go some way toward answering questions on the practical side, but funeral directors may also be relied upon to help and give support. They are always sympathetic and may be contacted at any time, either before or after registration of the death. Some people even make arrangements for their own funeral with a funeral director. They are often on call 24 hours a day, which is especially comforting when a death occurs at home. I shall concentrate on the practical problems following adult death; those following perinatal death have been reviewed recently by Forrest *et al.* (1981).

(a) Registration

When a patient dies, the doctor who has been looking after him fills in a 'Medical Certificate of Cause of Death', commonly called the 'death certificate.' This asks for certain simple information; the name and age of the patient, the date and place of death, the date last seen alive and the cause of death. Exceptions to this general rule are discussed under 'The coroner' below.

There is a statutory requirement for the doctor to have seen the patient for the condition causing death within two weeks before death, but no obligation by law to see the body after death. Doctors are expected to be as accurate as possible, not only to prevent concealment of crime, but also to provide accurate statistical information.

The certificates are supplied by the registrar of births and deaths in books of fifty, with counterfoils. Each completed certificate has two parts: the main portion, which is sealed in an envelope addressed to the registrar, and a detachable portion; the 'Notice to Informant', which is usually pinned to the outside of the envelope. This carries a list of people qualified to inform the registrar of the death (that is, to register the death) and also a list of particulars about the deceased which the informant should be able to give the registrar.

These are:
1. The date and place of death, and the deceased's usual address.
2. Deceased's full name (and maiden name if a married woman or widow).
3. Date and place of birth.
4. Occupation (and that of her husband if the deceased was a married woman or a widow).
5. Whether in receipt of a pension or an allowance from public funds.
6. If married, the date of birth of the surviving spouse.

The deceased's medical card should also be delivered to the registrar.

The informant usually takes the certificate to the registrar and registers the death. This takes about thirty minutes, and the informant signs the entry in the register. The registrar then issues the 'Certificate of Registration of Death' (similar to the birth and marriage certificates) and gives the informant copies if he should need them (for banks, insurance companies and so on). He also supplies the necessary forms for claiming the death grant (currently £30 for adults) and issues a slip, 'Certificate for Disposal after Registry'. This is sufficient authority for burial, but further certificates are needed for cremation (see below). The informant then takes the Certificate for Disposal to a funeral director and makes the arrangements for the funeral.

It is interesting to note that we have no say in law in what happens to our bodies. Even a wish expressed in a will is not binding on the executor, nor does carrying a kidney donor card oblige the next of kin to offer organs for transplantation. They do, however, make one's wishes known, and these are usually respected. The exception to this rule is that if the deceased has previously forbidden cremation in writing, or verbally to two persons, he may not be cremated.

The first cremation in a public crematorium in England took place in Woking in 1885. Since then the practice has become widespread, and now the majority of people dying in a large city are cremated. The regulations governing cremation are based on those which the Cremation Society formulated in the nineteenth century.

Several forms have to be completed before a cremation can take place. Form A is supplied to the funeral director by the crematorium. It constitutes an

*Reprinted with kind permission from *Nursing Times,* March 17th, 463–464, 1982.

application for cremation and is filled in by the executor. It includes questions as to whether close relatives have been informed of the proposed cremation, and whether they have expressed any objection. The funeral director will then ask the general practitioner or hospital for the medical certificates (Forms B and C). The first of these is completed by the patient's medical attendant, usually the doctor who signed the 'Medical Certificate of Cause of Death'. Form C is filled in by another practitioner who has been qualified for at least five years, and is not related to, nor a partner of, the first. Both doctors must see and identify the body, and answer various questions as to the time, cause, and mode of death, names of persons present at the time of death, etc.

The documents are sent to the medical referee of the crematorium, who alone is able to authorise cremation, which he does by signing form F (B, C and F are on one piece of paper). Forms D and E are for use by the coroner, but the medical referee must still authorise cremation. After the cremation, the particulars are entered in a Register of Cremations (Form G).

(b) Costs

Funeral directors' fees for a funeral providing one car and veneered coffin are in the range £200–£250. A solid coffin may add up to £100 to this figure (south London prices, 1981). Additional fees may be incurred depending on whether the service is followed by cremation or a burial. Fees for a cremation total £78 at the time of writing: in the case of a burial the cost of the grave is very variable (£200 upwards in south London) and the cost of a stone will again add £200–£400. Fairly typical minimum costs would therefore be £300 for a cremation, £650 for a burial. The cost of the funeral is of course recoverable from the estate after probate.

(c) The coroner

The law appears to require doctors to complete a 'Medical Certificate of Cause of Death' in all cases. In certain circumstances there is a statutory requirement for the registrar to inform the coroner of a death. Some of these are:

(i) When the doctor has not seen the patient within fourteen days of death.
(ii) When the doctor has not truly been in attendance. A doctor is not usually considered to have been in attendance unless he has examined the patient on two occasions. In practice, in hospitals an admission lasting less than 24 hours would be reported to the coroner.
(iii) When the patient has died of an industrial disease.
(iv) When violence, accident, neglect or poisoning has contributed to the death.
(v) When death has occurred during an operation or before recovery from an anaesthetic.

It is, however, widespread practice for the medical attendant to report deaths in the above categories without writing a certificate. The coroner acts through his officer, a member of the police force, who makes enquiries of the family and doctor on the coroner's behalf. He may decide, if the doctor is confident of the cause of death, to waive the coroner's interest, so that the normal procedure of certification applies. This is a favour granted to doctors in order to protect bereaved relatives from distressing enquiries and possibly delay, and should not be abused. If the coroner's officer accepts the case, he makes his enquiries, and orders a post-mortem. An inquest only takes place in cases of unnatural death. A coroner's post-mortem may delay a funeral by up to a week.

(d) Other post-mortems

Most hospital post-mortems are requested in order to obtain the answer to a specific question: 'What is the precise diagnosis?' 'What is the extent of the disease?' 'How has our treatment modified the disease?' or 'Why were this patient's symptoms difficult to control?' If a post-mortem is thought desirable, the doctor concerned should ask the next of kin and must obtain written consent. Depending on how much information is needed, so the thoroughness of the examination will vary, but most post-mortems are not markedly disfiguring, and should not delay funeral arrangements. They are also an invaluable means of learning new possibilities in any medical field. Ultimately most knowledge of the natural history of diseases rests upon a full understanding of their pathology.

(e) Transplantation

Tissue transplantation is a widespread and valid method for treatment of several chronic conditions, and is sometimes the only means available. The easiest tissue to transplant is the cornea. This is because the cornea has no blood supply and therefore survives as viable tissue for a relatively long time after death. Its avascularity also means that tissue typing is unnecessary, and rejection is uncommon. Corneal grafts are used to restore sight in patients whose own corneas have become opaque through scarring. Naturally, before any tissue can be given the next of kin's written consent must be obtained.

Other organs may be transplanted (some commmonly some, as yet, experimentally), including kidneys, livers and hearts. Other possibilities could include pancreas and lung. Here, however, the situation is more complicated because:

(i) The transplant recipient will take immuno-suppressive drugs to prevent rejection, so, that any possibility of infection or malignant cells in the donor's blood or the organ itself prevents its use.

(iii) Without their blood supply, these organs only remain viable for a short time unless stored in ice. This means that the donor must be maintained on a ventilator until immediately before removal of the organs. This period allows clinical tests for brain death to be applied (Conference of Medical Royal Colleges, 1976). Despite recent controversy, these appear to be very reliable, Editorial (1981).

These factors greatly limit the numbers of potential donors and the great majority are previously healthy people who die in hospital of a brain tumour, head injury or massive stroke.

In all of the above, we must remember that our first concern should be to deal sympathetically with bereaved relatives. It helps if we can be efficient and provide order and structure for relatives. The procedures described may be commonplace to us, but many people have no knowledge of how a funeral is arranged, and we should take care that they understand what is the next step. In asking permission for a post-mortem or donation of organs, all the staff involved should be honest about what will happen, so that relatives can understand why we ask their permission, but we must not be over-persuasive. They have many things to worry about, and are often reluctant to give their permission for such things, but this may be overlaid by a wish not to appear mean. Often they find the answer by asking themselves. 'What would he have wanted?'

References

Conference of Medical Royal Colleges and their Faculties in the United Kingdom, Diagnosis of brain death, *Br. med. J.*, **2**, 1187–1188, 1976

Editorial, Brain death, *Lancet*, **1**, 363–365, 1981

Forrest, G.C., Claridge, R.S. and Baum, J.D., Practical management of perinatal death, *Br. med. J.*, **282**, 31–32, 1981

Further reading

Earle, A. M., Argondizzo, N. T. and Kutscher, A. H., *The Nurse as Caregiver for the Terminal Patient and his Family*, Columbia University Press, 1976

Hector, W. and Whitfield, S., *Nursing Care for the Dying Patient and the Family*, Heinemann, 1982

Hinton, J., *Dying*, Penguin, 1971

Lamerton, R., *Care of the Dying*, Penguin, 1980

Mansell Pattison, E., *The Experience of Dying*, Prentice Hall, 1977

Parkes, C. M., *Bereavement*, Penguin, 1975

Polson, G. J. and Marshall, T. C., *The Disposal of the Dead*, 3rd edn, English Universities Press, 1975

Ross, E. K., *The Experience of Dying*, Tavistock, 1973

Sampson, C., *The Neglected Ethic: Religious and Cultural Factors in the Care of Patients*, McGraw-Hill, 1982

Smith, K., *Help for the Bereaved*, Duckworth, 1978

Chapter 5   Pain

by Jennifer Raiman

For the happiness mankind gain
Is not in pleasure, but in rest from pain.

John Dryden (1631–1700)

Only pain is real, I'm not frightened to die, but for me pain is the only reality.

Woman 42 years old, Carcinoma breast with secondaries (1980)

Look at me, I've lost so much weight, I'm in so much pain, that even the pillows hurt me now — I need you to understand.

Man 56 years old, Carcinoma tongue with secondaries (1980)

Pain has always been part of our shared human experience, with complete congenital insensitivity to pain a rare phenomenon. For hundreds of years remedies have been sought and potions used, seeking to relieve pain, and its attendant suffering. The experience of pain is subjective, individual and private, and has been reflected and portrayed in works both of literature and art, from ancient civilisations to the present day. Historically it has been a subject for enquiry by diverse disciplines, philosophers, theologians, social anthropologists, physicians and in more recent years, nurses.

Theories of pain mechanisms

Theories to explain the mysteries of pain are continually undergoing rapid change as new evidence becomes available from research. Two major theoretical concepts of pain, the specificity and pattern theories, provide the basis of the varied approaches and controversies.

1   The specificity theory

Sinclair (1955) suggested that free nerve endings are pain receptors and generate pain impulses that are carried by delta and C fibres in peripheral nerves and by the spinothalamic tract, to a pain centre in the thalamus. He assumed that nerve endings in the skin took various forms that corresponded to a different sensation: touch, cold, heat and pain.

2   The pattern theory

Goldscheider (1894) and Livingstone (1943) first proposed that stimulus intensity and central summation are the critical determinants of pain and in 1965 'The Gate Theory' (Melzack and Wall, 1965) described a 'Gate Control' system modulating sensory input from the skin before it evokes pain reception and response. The more recent identification of the morphine-like substances endorphins and encephalins throughout the nervous system enables examination of the endplate biochemical mediation of painful sensation and the sites of action of analgesics in neurotransmitters. There is mounting evidence to suggest that encephalins are released during acupuncture and pain therapy involving electrical stimulation of the brain. This has led to the evolution of the more recent endogenous pain suppression theory. These fields of study are constantly expanding and changing as new evidence comes to light. There is, however, no one theory which can fully explain the phenomenon of pain.

Definition of pain

The word *pain* is derived from the Greek word *poiné* for penalty which instantly suggests the concept of punishment and retribution associated with some cultures — a feeling reflected by some religious beliefs, that suffering and pain enoble the spirit. In life some short-lived periods of pain experience are not only inevitable, they may serve to strengthen and formulate character. Conversely, unrelieved, protracted pain can become a nightmare world of helplessness and despair, that can destroy the quality of life.

Pain disables overall more people than any other single disease entity, and is the most compelling reason for a person to seek assistance (Zborowski, 1969). Patients with pain pose a special problem to the art and practice of nursing. Pain and suffering, like joy and happiness, are subjective abstractions. To encompass this challenge, nursing response must be informed, unprejudiced and sensitive to each individual patient. It must be free from misconceptions and rooted in the basic principle of acceptance, that there is no 'correct level of pain', the patient must be the arbiter of his/her pain.

Basic anatomical and physiological considerations in the sensation of pain

Pain perception is initiated by the stimulation of a receptor pain corpuscle in the periphery, at the beginning of a sensory nerve fibre (Figure 5.1).

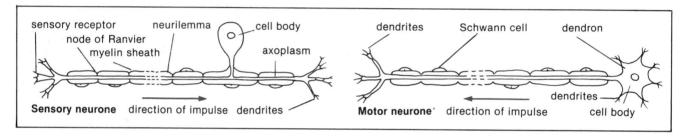

Figure 5.1   Sensory and motor neurones

(a) Sensory neurones

Pain starts as a chain impulse conducted along the axon as an electrical change of polarity within the fibre, changing from positive to negative by the movement across the semi-permeable membrane of sodium ions, surrounding potassium ions in the negative interior (Figure 5.2). This impulse enters the central

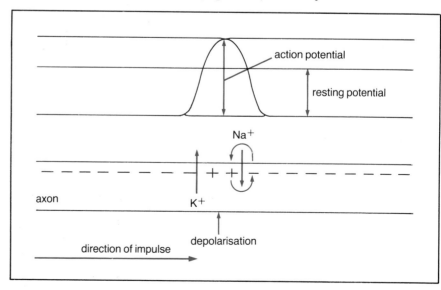

Figure 5.2   The passage of a nerve impulse

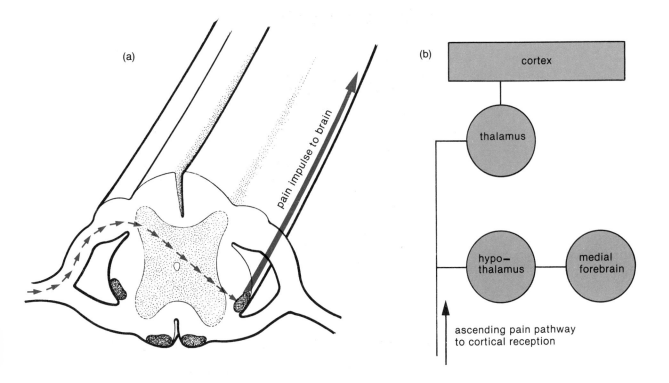

Figure 5.3 *Ascending brain pathways, (a) Cross section of spinal cord and (b) diagrammatic pain pathway*

nervous system (Figure 5.3) via the dorsal root ganglion, the dorsal root, across the dorsal horn to the opposite spinothalamic tract, and ascending through the medulla and pons (medial leminiscus) to be relayed in the thalamus, and thence via the internal capsule to the appropriate sensory cortex in the cerebral hemisphere.

Thus pricking your right index finger will be perceived at the post central gyrus of your left cerebrum (Figure 5.4).

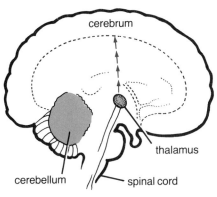

Figure 5.4 *Perception of pain impulses*

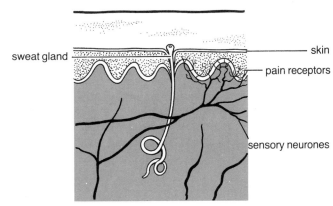

Figure 5.5 *Subcutaneous pain receptors*

(b) Pain receptors

The cross section biopsy of skin surface shows the distribution of pain receptors (Figure 5.5). The nerve endings present can be seen as free terminals in the layer. In some areas of the body the only sensation transmitted is pain. However, in other parts, for example in the cornea where the nerve endings are likewise seen as free terminals, cold, heat, touch and pain are all felt. To date it has not been possible to identify any one particular receptor uniquely associated with pain. Free nerve endings respond very differently in respect to threshold behaviour, adaption and frequency of response firing to stimuli.

The most basic response to pain is the primitive 'withdrawal reflex'. For example when touching a hot object the hand is withdrawn immediately. This is an involuntary response and does not involve the complex components of perception.

(c) Referred pain

This is a phenomenon of imperfect localisation and interpretation probably occurring at the spinal level. This confusion and misinterpretation in the cerebrum arises as the nerves from both visceral and somatic structures enter the central nervous system at the same level and share the same ascending pathways. Pain arising from structures deep in the body, for example the heart, occurs at the site of the organ and as 'referred pain' some distance away. Patients with acute coronary pain may complain of pain in the chest of a crushing nature together with severe gripping pain in the left arm. Referred pain associated with visceral disease may be indicative of extensive tissue damage and may herald a stage of advanced disease. The phenomenon of referred pain is consistent and therefore has considerable value in diagnosis. It can also produce 'trigger points' when the skin of an area to which pain is referred becomes particularly sensitive. If subjected to pressure these trigger points will produce pain in the referred areas and at the original pain site.

(d) Summary of relationships in pain perception (Figure 5.5)

This illustrates the relationship between events in pain perception, and the responses to the experience of pain (derived from correlations between neurophysiological mechanisms and psychological observations on the dimensions of pain experience) (Loeser, 1980; Melzack and Denis, 1978; Littlejohn and Vere, 1981).

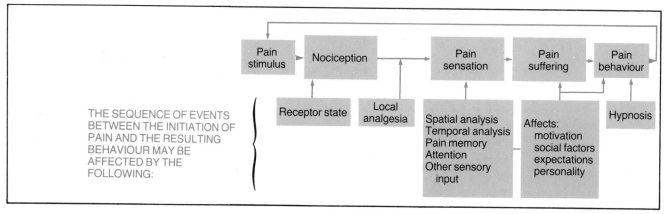

Figure 5.6   Pain sensation

After a *pain stimulus* occurs it passes into the receptor state or *nociception* (Figure 5.6). This is where unpleasant (noxious) stimuli are detected by receptors and converted into impulses carried by small fibre (A and C) afferent nerves to the cortex, where it is analysed as a *pain sensation*. At this stage the perception of pain will depend on the individual's interpretation of it. This will be expressed interms of distress, *pain suffering* which will determine *pain behaviour*, i.e. individual response to pain.

(e) Summary

1. The experience of pain is not a simple straightforward response to an unpleasant sensation. It is a highly complex event involving many nerve pathways and mechanisms.
2. At its most basic level it can be an immediate involuntary response disassociated from the complexities of perception and reaction.
3. Perception and response are dependent on other sensory inputs, motor activity, emotional state and past memory (Figure 5.7).

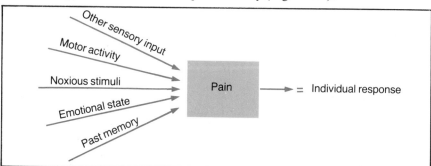

Figure 5.7   The elements of pain

Nursing response

To respond effectively to pain, goals need to be set and care planned individually. Additional inter-related components must be taken into account, that actively reflect patients' needs. Listening to patients provides the link, together with factors that influence response to pain:

1. Physical and pathological causes of pain (Figure 5.8).
2. Factors influencing response to pain (Figure 5.9).
3. Factors which modify the pain threshold (Figure 5.10).
4. Common symptoms which influence the response to pain (Figure 5.11).
5. Characteristics and differences between acute and chronic pain (Table 5.1).

> **Patient's comments:**
>
> 'Look at me, I've lost so much weight, I'm in so much pain that even the pillows hurt me now — I need you to understand.'
>
> *A man, 55 years old, cancer of the tongue with secondaries.*

Reactions to pain will vary between individuals. Some patients may accept pain and illness and evolve their own ways of coping.

> **Patient's comments:**
>
> 'I ignore it to a degree to handle it — pain well one almost becomes adjusted to it. Although I mind about the pain, and being ill, I handle it by fighting. In that way I reduce it to an irritant to my existence. I don't dwell on it.'
>
> *A man, 42 years old, Ankylosing Spondylitis.*

Some patients may become depressed and withdrawn; speaking little, sitting apart from others or lying on their beds.

> **Patient's comments:**
>
> 'I lie still and press the pillow into my stomach and close my eyes. I feel as if there is nothing left for me. I'm locked into my own world. I don't speak to anyone, and no-one speaks to me.'
>
> *A woman, 63 years old, Colonic cancer.*

Fear and anxiety enhance the perception of pain and intensify its severity. Pain is harder to bear in the absence of loved ones and friends. Or at night when sleep is poor and interrupted, combined with the normal ebbing of physiologic responses in the early hours with the lack of light and daytime activity.

> **Patient's comments:**
>
> 'Night's are bad, so bad for me, I lie here and it's just a different place to the day. Hearing people in pain, and my own twisting and gripping me, I fear the nights most of all. I try to lie still so as not to worry the nurses. I would like to go home, not just for the weekend but for keeps.'
>
> *A man, 69 years old, Bladder cancer.*

For some patients fear of the serious nature of an illness and the meaning of pain may lead to complete denial of both disease and the existence of pain.

> **Patient's comments:**
>
> 'I hid what I had from my husband for a whole year. I'm so frightened of what it means, I pretended it wasn't there.'
>
> *A woman, 42 years old, Stage IV Breast cancer.*

Fear and anxiety intensify pain, and patients who have experienced a long illness, a series of operations or long term distressing therapy, for example radiotherapy and cytotoxic drugs, may feel increasingly demoralised and experience mounting difficulties in contending with pain.

Some patients withdraw, others may call out, moan, weep, beg for help, become restless, pacing up and down, or toss and turn in bed or express thoughts of suicide.

- Infiltration of nerve, blood vessels and periosteum by tumour cells
- Compression of nerves by tumour mass
- Infection
- Inflammation and necrosis
- Ischaemia
- Distension of pelvic and abdominal viscera, lymphoedema
- Malignant ascites and effusion, elevated intracranial pressure
- Venous thrombosis and pulmonary embolism
- Ulceration

Figure 5.8   Physical and pathological causes of pain

- Genetic
- Personality
- Ethnic
- Cultural
- Environmental
- Experience
- Socio-economic

Figure 5.9   Factors influencing response to pain

Threshold lowered
- Insomnia
- Fatigue
- Anxiety
- Fear
- Anger
- Sadness
- Depression
- Mental isolation
- Introversion
- Past experience

Threshold raised
- Sleep
- Rest
- Sympathy
- Understanding
- Diversion
- Elevation of mood
- Analgesics
- Antidepressants

Figure 5.10   Factors which modify the pain threshold

- Anorexia
- General malaise and lassitude
- Constipation
- Diarrhoea
- Nausea and vomiting
- Cough
- Dyspnoea
- Inflammation
- Oedema
- Immobility
- Anxiety and fear
- Depression
- Dryness of the mouth and fungal infections

Figure 5.11   Common symptoms of disease which influence the response to pain

Whilst these may be recognised as individual reactions, cultural traditions and past environmental and parental attitudes will mediate response to pain. In general, Western culture does not encourage free expression of pain or emotion. Little children are discouraged from a very early age from crying and are told to be brave, whilst other cultures traditionally encourage a more spontaneous and open emotional response to life events.

It therefore seems reasonable that these differences in attitudes will not only influence behaviour to pain but exert an influence on its perception.

Likewise, these attitudinal differences and approach to pain will be present in staff. These will at times manifest themselves in day to day patient care. **It is implicit in caring for each patient to have due regard and countenance not only for what is familiar but equally to respect and have compassion for that which is not. Nursing has no brief for moral or cultural judgements.**

Differences between acute and chronic pain

These are shown in Table 5.1

Table 5.1*

	Acute pain	Chronic pain
Conduction pathways	Rapid	Slow
Tissue injury	Clearly causal	Minor or absent
Autonomic response	Present	Absent
Biological value	High	Low
Mood	Anxiety	Depression, anxiety
Social effects	Slight	Marked
Effective treatment	Analgesics	Variable, sometimes none

* Data after Twycross (1976).

Whether pain is acute or chronic care must be balanced in three areas: (1) Physical; (2) psychological; (3) social.

Physical care enhanced by a knowledge of both social and psychological factors is important.

In acute pain of limited duration the social effects are slighter, but studies have assessed the effect of education and encouragement on patients admitted for curative surgery. Results showed that the post-operative analgesics required were half that of a control group and that they were discharged three days earlier.

Chronic pain has been described graphically (Twycross, 1976):

'as a situation rather than an event'.

Unlike acute pain that has a meaning where its presence can be seen as a signal or warning that prompts action and remedial relief, unrelieved continuous pain is intensified by its lack of meaning and it becomes a threat not only to the patient's everyday living, but in the end is seen as a threat to life itself.

> **Patient's comments:**
>
> 'The pain never ceases, it is constant like a generator hammering and hammering. I have been taken over and destroyed by pain, I cannot now remember my life without pain'.
>
> *A woman, 66 years old, Breast cancer with secondaries.*

With anticipation of patients' needs and attention to factors that can modulate pain threshold (*see* figures 5.8–5.10), combined with thoughtful planned care, much can be done, not only to alleviate pain but to improve the quality of patients' day to day living, both in hospital and at home in a practical way.

For example:
- Heat pads carefully positioned.
- Cold packs for headaches.
- Warm baths — aid relaxation and ease tension.
- Meticulous attention to mouthcare (crushed ice to suck, warm gargles, lipsalve for cracked lips).
- Abdominal distension due to flatus relieved by enema or rectal tube.

- Bladder distension — catheterisation.
- Listening to patients, demonstrating continuing concern will not only support them but actively ease feelings of anxiety and depression, that increase pain.
- Careful planning of medication is needed to avoid necessary pain occurring *before* any procedure. Turning and washing can cause great pain and distress. Skill and adequate help is needed to avoid this.
- Careful general positioning of the body before turning, with particular support to painful areas.
- Careful positioning of pillows.
- Additional support, for example immobilisation by collar, splints or traction.
- Additional aids for comfort:
  Sheepskin pads.
  Ripple mattress.
  Rubber rings.
  Bedrest.
  Cradle.
- Special beds will assist movement with minimal handling and will lessen both pain and distress.

(a) Pain in terminal illness

> 'I shall live a year barely longer. During the year, let as much as possible be done.'
>
> *Joan of Arc.*

In the twentieth century developments in health education and disease prevention, together with scientific discovery have greatly improved health care and life expectancy.

Medical and surgical advances in the past fifty years in particular combined with the advent of antibiotics, the development and use of radiotherapy and chemotherapeutic agents in malignant disease have dramatically altered the prognosis of previously fatal illnesses. In consequence death has become less acceptable to us all and has given rise to a philosophy in which death for some has no place. Pain at death is not inevitable and if present can in all but a few patients be well controlled.

No doubt there are many reasons why some patients die with pain uncontrolled. Sudden traumatic deaths, people dying in the prime of life and death in the young may be particularly hard to bear and understand. Some reasons rest with staff who become confused and negative in the face of death, subconsciously convinced that in some way death in itself is their failure — however, death for us all is inevitable. These reactions lead staff to adopt negative attitudes. Thus the planned analytical approach to care accepted and necessary and in all other clinical practices is not maintained and relief of pain is not set as an imperative goal, and patients suffer.

Patient's comments

As I can't be cured, in their minds they have dismissed me.
A woman, 39 years old, cervical cancer; multiple secondaries; intractable pain

Care for dying patients with pain is perhaps one of the most demanding tasks nurses must face. It is perhaps here particularly that the interactions of the physical and psychological needs already described summate.

(b) Talking to patients with pain

The expression of pain is shared by culture and developed by the society in which we live.

Direct conversation with patients is the most obvious form of communication. However, between 70% and 90% of communication by both patients and staff is non-verbal. Communication involves not only speech but sensitivity and alertness to the non-verbal cues of behaviour, posture and expression. For example, the following may be observed.

- Changes in normal behaviour.
- Marked withdrawal and/or depresssion.
- Restlessness and/or agitation.
- Clenching of fists or teeth.
- Facial grimacing.

- Strained drawn expression.
- Sallow or greyish facial colour.
- Sweating, cold and clammy skin.
- Loss of appetite.
- Rejection of company.
- Excessive fatigue and lassitude.

(c) The role of staff

Talking to patients can best be done by helping patients to relax, by sitting quietly and being ready to listen. Being seen to be 'busy' not only increases anxiety but results in poor if not failure of contact.

> **Patient's comments**
>
> 'The doctors and nurses are always rushing in and out, I want to tell them how I feel — but they say wait a minute I'll come back — but they never do, I just seem to miss out all the time.'
> *A man, 35 years old, Lymphoma.*

Alternatively, persistent questioning and an 'inappropriate breeziness' in manner without giving time for answers stultifies response, manipulates the conversation, and inhibits further discussion. This serves only the staff, who by their actions keep all contact at their most superficial level and hasten away to the next problem and patient. This behaviour thwarts and blocks the creation of the right atmosphere in which trust and rapport can be established. For example:

A dying patient in pain will need encouragement to speak openly of fears that the pain will not become too great a burden to bear before he can receive the necessary reassurance and comfort.

A young mother admitted for emergency surgery leaving small children in the care of others needs time to share her problems.

The middle aged man with angina fearful for his job and future with the financial burdens of a family and mortgage to maintain, needs time to share his anxieties and fears.

Nurses are with patients for longer periods of time than any other member of the team. This unique situation for sustained contact, not only gives a greater opportunity to understand patients' problems but the additional responsibility of using this knowledge both sensitively and practically, by involving the skills of other people, e.g. physiotherapist, social worker, occupational therapist, chaplain.

(d) The family

Family and friends will need reassurance and the nurse can only anticipate the patient's needs but understand and support the family.

Being 'busy' increases anxiety and tension and will result in impoverished contact. Prompt attention to the patient will help to reduce the level of anxiety.

However, staff and family may communicate their worry and concern to the patient and thus by lowering his threshold increase distress and pain.

> **A relative's comments**
>
> 'Pain that is uncontrolled leads to a death without dignity. It destroys the person who suffers it, breaks the family who witness it and brands the staff that pass by on the other side.'
> *Mother of a dying patient.*

Some families are able to talk openly and support one another, but others become locked in their own private worlds of misery, unable to speak to each other, or to staff.

> **Patient's comments**
>
> 'No I don't talk to my husband, I don't say much — neither of us do, never have done really — it just seems to have got worse now.'
> *A woman, 58 years old, Breast cancer.*

Appreciation of the families relationships will add dimension and depth to the care of patients with pain.

Summary of general principles

- Pain is detrimental.
- Pain has physical, psychological, social and environmental components.
- Acute and chronic pain require different treatment approaches.
- Unrelieved pain creates a vicious circle, with anxiety, depression and fear; and it isolates. This may lead staff to avoid contact with the patient, at a time when the need for reassurance, comfort and positive action are increasing.
- The experience of pain is individual with no known 'correct levels' of intensity, suffering or response to treatment. The 'between patient' response can also be reflected as a 'within patient reaction', i.e. an individual patient's ability to respond and contend with pain will alter and change from time to time. The intensity levels of pain may also vary considerably during the day and night.

(a) Conclusion

Pain is a dual phenomenon

1. Perception of the sensation.
2. Emotional reaction to the sensation.

Affected by:

1. Cultural attitudes and values.
2. Past experience.
3. Present physical, emotional and mental states.

(b) Nursing role

Pain is a nursing responsibility and nurses can play a major role in its relief.
   This involves a dual responsibility:
   1. Planning and evaluating nursing care.
   2. Observing and reporting on the effects of treatment and care prescribed by others.

Effective management requires knowledge on:
   1. Mechanisms of pain.
   2. Site and severity of pain(s), including information of pain severity both at rest and on movement.
   3. Diurnal variation in the pain.
   4. The effect of analgesia.
   5. Other measures taken to relieve pain, i.e. lifting, repositioning, turning, massage, heat pads, additional aids, distracting activities, etc.
   6. Assessment — systematising and regularly monitoring the severity and relief of pain of the patient with a pain observation chart (Raiman, 1981) can be an effective way of caring.

(c) Adjuvant care

This consists of providing a positive supportive environment, free from disturbing stimuli, e.g. bright lights and excessive noise. It is essential to understand the value of other sensory inputs. When pain dominates, it will occupy the patient's complete attention. Providing and understanding the need for other distraction such as company, conversation, books, radio and television not only simply 'passes the time', but decreases pain and assists in its control by the diminution of its perception.

   Adequate sleep at night and the provision for specific rest periods during the day is important and tends to be overlooked. Poor quality sleep interrupted by pain leaves patients exhausted, demoralised and depressed. A good night's sleep enables the patient to contend more effectively with illness and pain during the day.

A nurse's presence can bring comfort and support. Sitting with patients, touching, holding hands, demonstrates care and concern and can effectively lessen the impact of pain.

Analgesia

The word analgesic is derived from two Greek words, *AN*—WITHOUT, and *ALGOS*—PAIN. Pain is a symptom not a disease and the type of treatment chosen will be dependent on two main factors:

1. Is the aim to give relief during and until the condition is investigated and treated?
2. Or in chronic conditions, e.g. arthritis, or malignant disease, when 'to cure' is not a practical or feasible goal, to achieve and maintain good pain control?

Analgesic medications are among the most usual methods used to relieve pain. Whilst the initial responsibility for prescribing is medical, the nursing roles of (1) administration and observation; and (2) assessment and reporting the efficacy of analgesia prescribed, are both essential and mutually complementary.

Nurses are with their patients for longer periods of time than other members of the team. This offers a unique opportunity to participate actively in the use of analgesics. To achieve this goal, judgement must be exercised; for example, if more than one analgesic is prescribed or a range of dose is available, these responsibilities assume: (1) A depth of knowledge on how analgesics work and their potential side effects; (2) the ability to judge and assess individual patient's needs and response.

Pain is rarely a static state. Patients need to be assessed individually and regularly throughout each 24-hour period.

1 Assessment

Analgesic relief should be assessed in relation to comfort achieved:
1. at night;
2. during the day and at rest;
3. on movement.

2 Reassessment

This is needed, particularly for patients with chronic multifocal pain. 'Old pains may get worse, and new ones emerge.' Review is essential.

3 Evaluation

This is regular, detailed evaluation on the efficiency of analgesics following administration, as follows:

1. How long does it take for the drugs to work?
2. How much relief is achieved?
3. How long does the relief last?
4. Be alert for side effects.
5. Observe and report accurately.

4 Patient participation

This should be: (1) encouraged; (2) sought; (3) respected.

Definition

Analgesics are drugs that abolish or lessen pain, without causing a loss of consciousness.

Medications for the relief of pain have been known and their use documented for thousands of years. The perfect analgesic has yet to be discovered. However, there is a wide variety of compounds which whilst varying in their mode of action and potency, offer the ability to relieve pain.

Action of analgesics

Analgesics act upon the nervous system by affecting perceptual mechanisms. In addition narcotic drugs alter the emotional response to pain (cortical action). At the peripheral level the production of pain-producing substances in the tissues, such as kinins and prostaglandins, is interfered with by the use of salicylates, aspirin being the most common.

Classification of analgesics

To avoid confusion, it is helpful to consider analgesics in a graded table of efficacy.

Examples of analgesics:

MILD

Aspirin, paracetamol — non-narcotic.

MODERATE

Codeine, propoxyphene (dihydrocodeine), dipipanone (Diconal) — weak narcotic.

SEVERE

Diamorphine, morphine, levorphanol (Dromoran), methadone (Physeptone), phenazocine (Narphen) — strong narcotic.

(a) Analgesics: basic principles

It is essential to have a thorough understanding of the various types of analgesics and the basic principles underlying and governing their use, e.g.:

- Duration of action.
- Potency.
- Toxicity and side effects.
- Agonists and antagonists.
- Efficacy.
- Cumulation.
- Tolerance.
- Dependence.

Also needed is an appreciation that chronic pain needs regular analgesia, e.g. each dose is given before the pain returns; 'as required' prescribing is not compatible with protracted pain, except to make available additional adjuvant analgesics to boost and enhance the regular doses.

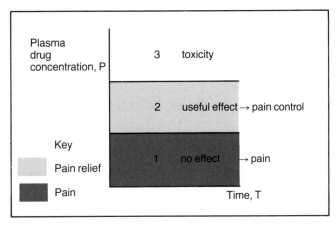

Figure 5.12 Plasma concentration zone in relation to drug effects.
This is also the key to Figures 5.13 to 5.17

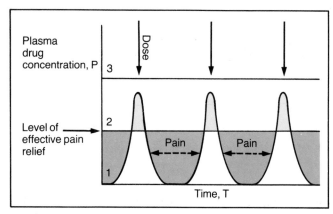

Figure 5.13   *Short-acting drugs*

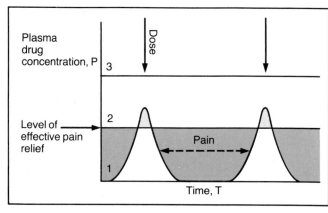

Figure 5.14   *Overspaced doses or 'as required' analgesia*

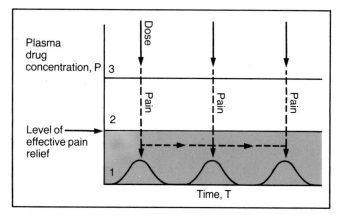

Figure 5.15   *Doses too small to achieve pain relief. N.B. Giving analgesia does not automatically produce pain relief*

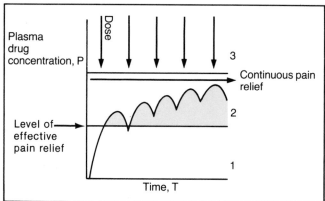

Figure 5.16   *Doses spaced at satisfactory intervals to maintain analgesia. In chronic pain (such as in cancer) analgesia must be given regularly throughout the 24-hour period to achieve continuous pain relief*

Note: See Figure 5.12 for key to these figures.

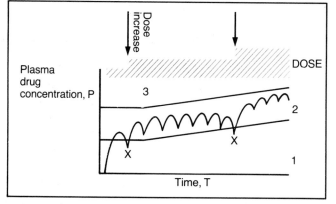

Figure 5.17   *The effects of tolerance. Dosage is increased at X to maintain pain control as tolerance occurs*

1   Individual variation

There is a wide range of individual variation at any age, but particularly sensitive are the very young or older patients.

2   Duration of action

Drugs vary in length of time within which they act, i.e. remain effective. For example, morphine and diamorphine are short acting drugs, the half-life of their analgesic effect is between two and four hours. This follows closely the plasma drug concentration. The aim is to maintain the plasma level of the analgesic in the therapeutic 'useful effect' band but below that of toxicity.

3   Efficacy

This is the maximum effect a given dose will produce. In severe pain only opiates and opioids have sufficient efficacy.

4   Potency

This is a comparison of dose (milligram to milligram) between two similarly acting drugs. Therefore increasing the dose beyond a certain level does not improve potency.

5   Toxicity

This is a level at which drugs cause unwanted effects, for example, aspirin can cause tinnitus and opiates respiratory depression.

6   Cumulation

This is the gradual build up and storage of a drug in the tissues. For example, the metabolism of methadone is complex and it has a far longer half-life than that of morphine or diamorphine and remains in the body for a greater period.

7   Tolerance

This occurs when the body becomes used to a drug and a larger dose is needed to maintain pain relief. Fortunately, this does not inevitably produce toxicity, for if tolerance occurs the level at which side effects become a problem rises in proportion.

8   Dependence

Physical dependence will develop with patients receiving opiates and opioids, i.e. drugs that exhibit tolerance also produce dependence. This is not the same as addiction which has a very strong link with drug abuse and a psychological component. Even after long term use opiates can be tapered off and withdrawn if this is clinically appropriate.

9   Agonists, partial agonists, antagonists

Opiate and opioid drugs differ in their affinitive to bind with the opiate receptors in the brain.

Pure agonists   — morphine and diamorphine.
Partial agonists   — pentazocine and codeine.
Antagonists   — naloxone and naltroxone.

These give very basic facts about a series of highly complex mechanisms. In practical terms, using a mixture of pure agonists with partial agonists will decrease analgesic effect, whilst antagonists will reverse the action of pure agonists (which whilst preventing pain relief can be used to reverse the side effects of respiratory depression).

10   Neurosurgical measures

Unrelieved 'intractable pain' such as the pain of nerve compression and infiltration may be helped by neurosurgical techniques, such as:

1. Rhizotomy (nerve blocks) blocks the pain before the sensory route enters the spinal cord.
2. Cordotomy, in which sensory pathways in the spinal cord are cut, relieves pain below the operative site.
3. Dorsal column stimulators — these are surgically implanted in the spinal column.
4. Transcutaneous nerve stimulators — worn externally (battery controlled) and can be switched on-off by the patient (stimulator acts by altering or blocking pain with alternative stimulation).

11   Additional techniques to relieve pain

The development of new techniques such as relaxation and imagery is aimed at lessening the perception of pain by encouraging the patient to become skilled in the use of relaxation to decrease stress. In imagery the patient uses the imagination to develop pleasant sensory images to decrease the perception of pain, these may be linked with bio-feedback techniques and hypnosis.

Attitudes to pain

The goals of individualised care and management of pain must involve a close nurse/patient relationship. Examination and understanding of both personal and collective professional attitudes, values and beliefs in response to pain and its assessment are essential.

Summary

Patients do not cease to exist as individuals because of pain and illness; nor do they become a collection of signs and symptoms, to be dealt with in isolation, e.g. 'the stomach cancer in bed 3 with secondaries'.

As individuals, patients have the right to have their wishes listened to and respected.

When illness and pain make independent thought and action difficult they have the right to receive care compatible with the maintenance of human dignity.

Patients have the right to be believed.

A note on the recording of pain

Pain is a wholly subjective symptom, In consequence, there is no easy way of understanding what a patient is suffering, nor of conveying information about it from one person to another, though doctors and nurses need to do so. For instance, a doctor who needs to check the effectiveness of an analgesic prescription may find it difficult to say what information should be decisive. Thus, problems of communication can result in poor control of pain.

(a) The London Hospital pain observation chart

First, the pain observation chart used at The London Hospital is intended to improve communication between nurse and patient by making the recording of pain more systematic; the idea owes a lot to charts for neurological observations. Secondly, it is intended to make readily available in one place the

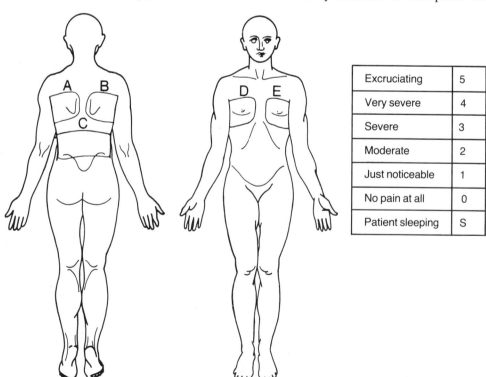

Excruciating	5
Very severe	4
Severe	3
Moderate	2
Just noticeable	1
No pain at all	0
Patient sleeping	S

Figure 5.18   Body outlines and severity scale

information that is useful when taking decisions about the management of pain; for this reason some information already available on the drug chart, and some in the nursing record, is inevitably duplicated in it. Thirdly, it is intended to focus attention on the mechanisms of different pains, and to provide evidence on what relieves them, by recording each site of pain separately.

You are likely to find this chart most useful when you know that a patient's pain is a problem, or you think it may be. It is a means of communication, to be used *with* the patient, not *on* the patient. Nurses should have it available at the handover report between shifts, and doctors will need it for ward rounds. The brief comments allowed may prove unexpectedly significant, and need amplification, so it is important that each entry is initialled. Occasionally, it may be a good idea to have two separate, independent charts, one kept by the patient, the other by the staff.

Time	Pain rating — By sites A	B	C	D	E	F	G	H	Overall	Analgesic given (Name, dose, route, time)	Lifting	Turning	Massage	Distracting activities	Position change*	Additional aids*	Other*	Comments from patients and/or staff	Initials
2.30pm	1	1	1 (0)	0	0					—				✓	✓				
15.30	1	1	3	1	1					—								Prepared for treatment	
18.00	1	1	2	0	0					—								DF 118 given at about 5pm but have little or no effect	
20.00	2	2	3	1	1					Pethidine (injection)					✓			Relief after about 20 mins	
15/4/82 04.30	0	0	2	0	0					Pethidine (injection)								Pain only just noticable but getting worse	
11.30	1	1	2	1	1					—								Sent for X Ray	
1.00pm	2	2	3	1	1					Paracetamol (oral)					✓			Pain aggravated by transference from couch to chair at X Ray	
1.30pm	1	1	2	1	1					—								Paracetamol has had some effect but not much	
2.30pm	1	1	2	1	1					Oxycodone (anal)									
3.00pm	0	0	1	0	0					—					✓			Pain has almost completely gone	
10.00pm	1	1	2	1	1					Paracetamol and Oxycodone (anal)								Pain had just appeared but showed signs of getting worse	
10.30pm	0	0	0	0	0					—								Able to sleep very comfortably	
16/4/82 4pm	2	2	3	1	1					Oxycodone (anal)					✓			Pain getting worse	
4.30pm	0	0	0	0	0					—								Pain almost completely gone again	
11.30	1	1	2	1	1					Oxycodone (anal)				✓				Spent a very comfortable morning, almost completely pain free	
7.00	1	1	3	1	1					Oxycodone (anal)								Weekend leave, painkillers needed after journey	
8.00	1	1	1	1	1					—								Painkillers effective after 1/2 – 1 hour	
17/4/82 4.30	2	2	3	1	1					Oxycodone (anal)					✓			Position change helps but only for a short while	
5.15	1	1	1	1	1					—								Painkillers effective 45 mins comfortable but not completely gone	
6.00	1	1	1	1	1					Paracetamol (oral)									
6.30	0	0	1	1	1					—								Paracetamol to relieve areas A & B slightly	
2.30pm	2	2	3	2	2					Oxycodone (anal)					✓			Position change helps but not much	

Measures to relieve pain (specify where starred)

Figure 5.19 Recording of pain and measures to relieve pain

The London Hospital
PAIN OBSERVATION CHART

This chart records where a patient's pain is and how bad it is, by the nurse asking the patient at regular intervals. If analgesics are being given regularly, make an observation with *each* dose and another *half-way between* each dose. If analgesics are given only 'as required', observe two-hourly. When the observations are stable and the patient is comfortable, any regular time interval between observations may be chosen.

To use this chart, ask the patient to mark all his or her pains on the body diagram below. Label each site of pain with a letter (i.e. A, B, C, etc).

Then at each observation time ask the patient to assess:

1. The *pain in each separate site* since the last observation. Use the scale above the body diagram, and enter the number or letter in the appropriate column.
2. The *pain overall* since the last observation. Use the same scale and enter in column marked *overall*.

Next, record what has been done to relieve pain. In particular:

3. Note any *analgesic* given since the last observation, stating name, dose, route and time given.
4. Tick any other *nursing care* or *action taken* to ease pain.

Finally note any *comment on pain* from patient or nurse (use the back of the chart as well, if necessary) and initial the record.

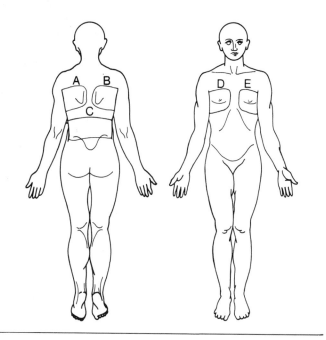

Date _____ Sheet number _____   Patient identification label

Time	Pain rating — By sites								Overall	Measures to relieve pain (specify where starred)										Initials
	A	B	C	D	E	F	G	H	Overall	Analgesic given (Name, dose, route, time)	Lifting	Turning	Massage	Distracting activities	Position change*	Additional aids*	Other*	Comments from patients and/or staff		

Adapted from the London Hospital Pain Observation Chart

Figure 5.20   The complete Pain Observation Chart. The reader will actually find the 'body diagram' referred to above on p. 76, and the 'scale' adjacent to it

References

Goldscheider, A., *Ueber den Schmerz in Physiologischer und Klinischer Milsicht,* Hirschwald, 1894

Littlejohn, D. W. and Vere, D. W., The clinical assessment of analgesic drugs, *Br. J. clin. Pharmacol.,* **11,** 319–332, 1981

Loeser, J. D., Perspectives on pain in clinical pharmacology and therapeutics, *Proceedings of the First World Conference* (ed. P. Turner), pp. 313–316, Macmillan, 1980

Melzack, R. and Dennis, S. G., Neurophysiological foundations of pain. In: *The Psychology of Pain* (ed. R. A. Sternbach), pp. 49–72, Raven Press, 1978

Melzack, R. and Wall, P.D., Pain mechanisms, a new theory, *Science,* **150,** 971, 1965

Raiman, J. A., Responding to pain, *Nursing,* Nov., 1362–1365, 1981

Sinclair, D. C., Cutaneous sensation and the doctrine of specific nerve energy, *Brain,* **78** (584), 1955

Sweet, W., Pain, *Handbook of Physiology,* Sect. 1, Vol. 1, Chapt. 19, pp. 459–506, 1959

Twycross, R., Relief of pain in advanced cancer, *Prescriber's Journal,* **18,** 117–124, 1978

Zborowski, M., *People in Pain,* Jossey-Bass, San Francisco, 1969

Further reading

The Dying Patient, CMF Publications, 1975. Twenty-two-page booklet on attitudes to the dying

Narcotic analgesics in terminal care, *Drugs and Therapeutics Bulletin,* **18,** 69–70, 1980

Hannington Kiff, J. G., *Pain Relief,* Heinemann, 1975

Hannington Kiff, J.G., *Pain Control,* South West Thames Cancer Service, 1976

Hayward, J., *Information — A Prescription Against Pain,* RCN, 1975

Hinton, J., *Dying,* Penguin Books Publication

Kubler-Ross, E., *On Death and Dying,* Tavistock Publications, 1970

McCaffery, M., *Nursing Management of the Patient with Pain,* Lippincott, 2nd edn, 1979

Parkes, C. M., *Bereavement,* Pelican Books, 1972

Sanders, C. M. (ed.), *The Management of Terminal Malignant Disease,* Arnold, 1978

Sternbach, R. A. (ed.), *The Psychology of Pain,* Raven Press, 1978

Chapter 6

Planning the nursing care of the patient

by Veronica Chapman

The qualified nurse today is being asked more and more to accept responsibility for independent thinking and action. This requires a high level of skill in collecting information from the patient and his family, adding to that information from the body of knowledge which the nurse herself possesses and finally planning the nursing care which truly supports that individual, and enables him to adapt to his illness. In other words the nurse must develop skills — becoming proficient in observation, data collecting, performing basic motor skills, and acquiring the ability to evaluate the results of her nursing actions. The ability to communicate not only with her patient, but with all those involved in the patient's care, is of the utmost importance and is central to the nurse's effective implementation of skilful and compassionate nursing care.

This part of the text is aimed at providing some tools for the nursing student or the nurse to use in order to make an accurate assessment of the patient's overall condition. However, in order to use the information that she has now collected effectively, a body of acquired knowledge is also necessary. An attempt will be made here to explore some normal behaviour needs and activities of daily living as a basis for comparison when a person becomes a patient or client. Many concepts will be dealt with to provide a broad base and references will be provided for the students who may wish to study a particular topic in greater depth. There will also be a recommended reading list. Although many patients and clients are cared for in a non-hospital setting, the major part of nursing training continues to take place in hospital so most concepts and techniques refer to the hospital environment, but they can easily be related to nursing care in the home.

Nursing must be considered in relation to the current overall concept of health care. The focus of the nurse within this framework is upon each patient and the process through which his individual needs can be met. Although most modern nursing literature reflects this approach to nursing care, the demonstration of the philosophy rests with each individual nursing student and nurse. The process of nursing (Yura and Walsh, 1978), is based on a problem-solving approach. This will be applied throughout the text. The four elements of the nursing process are the assessment stage, the identification of problems, the implementation of problem-solving strategies in the form of nursing care and evaluation of those strategies to ascertain their effectiveness. This process will be discussed in much greater depth at a later stage. It is the basic tool for devising a plan of care for each individual patient.

Health and illness

In an ideal world everyone should be in a state of good health. Increasingly this concept of health is being accepted as not only freedom from illness and disease but as a positive state of physical and mental well-being. This concept is often expressed as 'wellness', especially in American literature. It can be described as a condition of complete mental, physical, social and spiritual well-being which enables individuals to function in a normal manner to an optimum degree. Health can therefore be described as a dynamic state leading to physical and mental well-being and a state of general satisfaction with life.

The physiological condition of homeostasis which controls the internal environment of the body must also be included in this definition. The balance of this internal environment, and its constancy, is maintained by the interaction of all the systems of the body. When one of these systems ceases to function efficiently, there are built-in restorative mechanisms which come into play. If however, the imbalance is too great to be corrected, a state of illness may occur, requiring medical or surgical treatment.

Definition

Disease may be defined as a condition which reduces the normal functioning of an individual.

When psychological and social states of equilibrium are added to his physiological concept of homeostasis, then health, or 'wellness' is seen to require the maintenance of the person's:
(a) physiological balance;
(b) psychological and emotional balance;
(c) cultural and social balance;
(d) spiritual and philosophical balance.

Health care therefore involves not only the maintenance of efficient bodily functions, but the consideration and supervision of the individual interacting with his environment. Disorganisation of any of the above processes may lead to illness.

Sometimes, health and illness are regarded as being at opposite ends of a continuum with a number of intermediate stages.

(a) Stages along the good health–illness continuum

The nursing student should remember that it is the individual who actually determines when illness exists. She should therefore develop her awareness and understanding of the behaviour associated with ill health, as well as the physiological changes which may occur.

Beliefs and attitudes concerned with health are very personal in nature, and are often deeply rooted in the culture and customs of the society in which the person lives and has been educated. When a person feels well, he may engage in activities to prevent illness, to promote health, or to detect disease. Considerable emphasis is placed on this 'health behaviour' in some countries; jogging, 'health foods', exercise and fresh air, routine medical examination, cervical smears and self-examination of the breasts are examples of such behaviour.

When a person believes himself to be ill he engages in sick role behaviour. Falling ill is not something that happens to us — it is a choice we make as a result of the way we feel. In cases of emergency the individual's choice is minimal such as in cases of accident or sudden collapse, but these situations are rare. Most people who seek professional help have already taken on the role of patient, and as such begin to behave differently. They act out the sick role behaviour which is socially prescribed, and has cultural variations.

They may accept limitations imposed by the illness on personal choice and actions, and neglect duties which they might usually perform. The degree to which a person continues this behaviour depends on a number of factors which he will use to make decisions and choices. These include the visible nature of the illness; fear of the unknown; availability of professional assistance; the advice and opinions of those from whom help is sought; fear and anxiety about dependence and loss of control; the expectations of this episode especially with regard to previous experience of illness; and the function of 'significant others' such as family and close friends in the person's life. All of these perceptions are influenced by education, social status — occupation and income, attitudes to illness, personality, temperament and self-esteem.

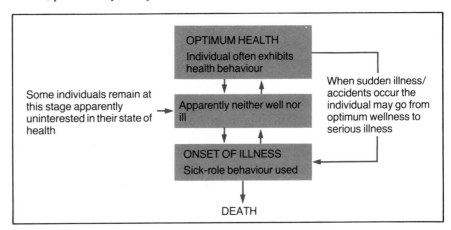

Figure 6.1   Stages along the continuum of health–illness

Models of nursing

(a) Physiological, psychological and social model

In order to cope with the health-illness continuum the person must successfully adapt to the constantly changing factors in his internal state and external environment. Coping mechanisms are largely physiological, psychological and social in origin. A model of nursing based on these principles has been developed by Calista *et al.*, 1974.

This model is based on the idea that human adaptation responses fall into four broad categories:

Physiological needs.
Self concept.
Role function.
Interdependence relations.

(b) Model based on the activities of daily living

Another model of nursing was described by Virginia Henderson, who gave 14 basic principles upon which nursing care is based. Nancy Roper *et al.* (1980) described The Activities of Daily Living (ADLs) which form the framework for assessment of the patient and his family and which correspond with Henderson's 14 principles.

In this text these models have been modified slightly in planning the patient's care using the nursing process based on a problem solving approach.

These 'activities of daily living' which may cause problems for the patient, where nursing support and intervention may be required are:

1. Breathing.
2. Eating and drinking.
3. Eliminating.
4. Maintaining a safe environment: physiological, psychological and social.
5. Communicating with others.
6. Expressing sexuality.
7. Personal cleansing and dressing.
8. Controlling body temperature.
9. Independent movement.
10. Working and playing.
11. Sleeping.
12. Dying.

None of these activities takes place in isolation. All are interdependent on some if not all the others. The patient's age is also a relevant factor, as he is constantly changing with advancing years, and each activity develops and changes with him. There are also continuums for each of the daily living activities. A person may be totally dependent or totally independent and the nurse's aim should be to assess the level of need accurately and to enable the patient to be as independent as possible.

1 Breathing

The process of breathing takes place in order to supply the body cells with oxygen, and to remove carbon dioxide. This is a vital function. If breathing ceases, irreversible damage to the neurones in the brain may occur within a few minutes.

The respiratory system is controlled by the respiratory centre in the medulla oblongata. This centre, with peripheral chemoreceptors in the arch of the aorta and in the carotid arteries controls the respiratory function, adjusting the rate and depth of respirations to meet the needs of the body. To do so, it responds to changes in the composition of the circulating blood's oxygen content (pO_2) and the arterial blood pressure together with neural activity initiated by stretch receptors in the lung tissue (Herring Brewer reflex).

In healthy individuals, and in patients whose illness does not affect the respiratory system, respirations are increased during exercise and by emotional factors such as excitement, anger and fear, when eating, and in extremes of body temperature. Voluntary control of breathing is possible for only a short period of time because the resulting chemical changes in the blood stimulate the respiratory centre which is more powerful in controlling breathing then the higher centres are.

2 Eating and drinking

The need for food, water and oxygen is common to all living organisms, and eating and drinking are vital for human survival. Disease and death are common in countries where adequate nutrition is impossible. The bodily changes occurring in starving individuals have been isolated and can be measured.

Food is used by the body for:

1. The production of energy for activity.
2. The structural repair (growth in children) of all cells.
3. The manufacture of substances such as enzymes and hormones.

A balanced diet contains carbohydrates, fats and proteins together with vitamins, minerals and trace elements. Most large hospitals employ dietitians for specific advice as well as aiding its overall menu planning, and nursing staff are encouraged to seek specialist support when problems arise.

Most people tend to prefer foods and eating patterns they learned as young children and may resist changing their established food habits. To most of us eating and drinking are enjoyable experiences.

In the western world as our way of life has changed over the years so we have developed and changed our nutritional patterns, which as a result has given rise to different nutritional problems. Fruits, vegetables and grain were the mainstay of most of the population at the beginning of the century, whereas now these are less predominant. Fat and sugar consumption has increased — probably to 50% of the total calorie intake per day. Alcohol consumption has increased — becoming a personal and social problem in many western countries.

Heart disease, cancer, cerebral-vascular disease, diabetes, atheroma, and cirrhosis of the liver are 6 of the 10 leading causes of death in the UK. Cholesterol, sugar, salt and alcohol have all been associated with the increasing incidence of such diseases — combined with stress factors and anxiety. The nurse plays an important part as a health educator, in advising others on the importance of a balanced diet.

3 Eliminating

The elimination of food and fluid waste products is closely related to the activities of eating and drinking. The body carries out this function in four different ways. The regulation of the amount of water contained in the body, together with the removal of the breakdown products of protein metabolism, is carried out by the kidneys, by the formation of urine.

Urine

The kidneys adjust the water balance of the body, and regulate the levels of mineral salts (often referred to as electrolytes) contained in the extracellular fluid, and the fluid within the body cells. In this way, the volume and concentration of the urine alters, according to the needs and activities of the body. The kidneys may also remove some poisons from the circulating blood, and they excrete some of the substances used in medication.

The urine formed by the kidneys is stored in the bladder, and the drive to urinate is triggered by the volume it contains. This process is reflex in infancy, but comes under voluntary control in healthy individuals through early training. Such control may be lost in certain diseases.

Perspiration and respiration

Water is also eliminated from the body in the form of water vapour during the process of respiration, and water and salts (mainly sodium chloride) are lost in the form of sweat, or perspiration. The amount excreted from the body by these two routes cannot be easily measured; it is referred to as 'insensible' loss. The environmental temperature and the size of the individual affect the amount lost by these routes. As a guide to this estimation, 500 ml is frequently used as the average loss for an adult when there is no significant rise in either the environmental or the body temperature. This should be taken into account when balancing the fluid intake and output.

A febrile (feverish) patient will lose more fluid by perspiration and respiration — when the loss of fluid through the skin is apparent — sensible loss is a term used to signify this.

Although elimination through the gastrointestinal tract is totally separate from that of the renal system, it can be influenced by lack of fluid which may lead to constipation. The upper part of the gastrointestinal tract is concerned with digestion and absorption of nutrients. The lower part, the colon, or large intestine is involved in the preparation of indigestible matter for elimination in the form of faeces and gases. The main function of the colon is in reabsorption of water and electrolytes and this function is affected by the general state of hydration of the body. A viscous alkaline mucus is secreted to facilitate the evacuation of faeces.

Defaecation

Faecal material is stored in the descending colon and when propulsed into the rectum the sensation to defaecate is experienced. Defaecation is also a reflex act in infancy which later comes under voluntary control. Elimination is usually practised in private and many strongly held attitudes have developed as a result of this. The digestive system is innervated by the autonomic nervous system, and is therefore affected by the emotional stress of illness, or by coming into hospital.

4 Maintaining a safe environment

In many ways, very little thought is given to the maintenance of a safe environment, since it is taken very much for granted.

When a person is ill, however, and particularly when he is admitted to hospital, many of the symbols of that safety are removed and he is required to adapt to unfamiliar patterns of behaviour and surroundings, and to a new routine in his activities of daily living.

Physiological safety

An individual may put a high value on his physiological safety, being very aware of his need for certain foods, for exercise, warmth and comfort, and cleanliness. He will be more threatened by changes in his pattern of living caused by disease or its treatment than another person who is less concerned with such values.

Psychological safety

People are protected by beliefs and attitudes which they share with others within a subcultural group. The culture concept is of very great importance and should never be underestimated. Everyone is part of one or more subcultures depending on occupation, income, religion and ethnic group. Custom and group habits are referred to as folkways and mores. Folkways are time honoured social habits that are often performed without thinking. Mores are customs that are regarded as particularly important and necessary for social welfare. They play an important part in the routine of daily living and carry an emotional impact that makes them resistant to change.

On a spiritual level a person's religious faith may also be of great importance to him on a day to day basis, enabling him to develop a supportive philosophy of life which leads to a high level of self-esteem.

At a personal level, human behaviour is strongly moulded by a territorial drive enabling the person to meet his needs of privacy, security, autonomy and identity.

Much has been written about personal space, and the feeling of discomfort experienced when other people come too close or establish unwelcome physical contact. The size of the personal space, the acceptance of touching, has marked variations in differing cultures, as well as varying between individuals. There are other effects of 'territorial behaviour', e.g. the elderly resident in a rest home, or the patient in a long stay unit, may always choose to occupy the same chair, and others may leave it vacant, even when she is not there. Another example is that of a nurse in a specialist area, who may feel threatened if her 'territory as an expert' is invaded — or when her expert knowledge is questioned — so that she responds defensively.

At times when it is not possible to keep a 'safe distance' from others, e.g. when travelling in a crowded vehicle, defensive behaviour may be observed by the avoidance of eye contact, reading a book, keeping arms close to the sides. If one is unable to control the proximity of strangers, the safest space to which one can retreat is to the centre of the body space, from here a sense of privacy can be retained by using non-verbal body cues to defend against intrusion.

Social safety

Safety in the home and in the community is important to most people — and rules for communal living are accepted when based on maintaining safety and security. Patients in hospital wards have to learn how to modify their activities for their own health — and for the needs of others, e.g. 'no smoking' areas are common, and noise and television may have to be reduced to meet the needs of others.

5   Communicating with others

The human need to communicate is universal. Even in babies who have died shortly after birth, the area of the brain known to be responsible for the generation of speech (Wernike's area) is found to be larger in the left hemisphere, in common with 98% of the population. This suggests the ability to speak is innate, and the fact that children appear to learn to speak relatively easily supports such a view.

Through language people express themselves in order to satisfy their needs and wishes, and are enabled to live with each other in a social order. When a person feels he has communicated his meaning to another person a feeling of satisfaction usually results. Effective communication is a two way process, resulting in personal growth and mutual understanding. Communication is both verbal — through speaking or the written word — and non-verbal, by eye contact, posture, expression, touch and the sharing of emotional responses.

Interpersonal relationships and the art of communication, should be developed through the nurse's professional career as they are at the heart of nursing in every setting.

6   Expressing sexuality

The sex of the individual is determined at conception. Men and women are brought up from childhood with different expectations and patterns of behaviour. Discussion about sexual differences, and about sexual intercourse has become more acceptable in recent times, and teaching of children in school has been extended to include some of the emotional aspects, and personal responsibility, as well as the biology of the sex organs. Many people, however, are embarrassed to discuss their thoughts and feelings about what it is to be a man, or to be a woman. At work or in social groups, people often behave differently to those of the opposite sex, than to those of the same sex. Expression of affection by physical contact in public is still considered by many people to be embarrassing and unnecessary. Whilst most adults show a preference to heterosexuality and much greater understanding of 'normal' sexual intercourse, and the physiological changes occurring in the woman's body as a result of the work by Masters and Johnson (1966), preference for homosexuality is probably more common that most people realise. The increase in understanding and acceptance of this in the UK may in part be due to the changes in a law relating to male homosexuality in the 1960s.

A nurse needs to be aware of the feelings of the patient in wards or units where both sexes are nursed together. The feelings of the individual person regarding privacy must be respected by the nurse — particularly in bathrooms, lavatories and in carrying out intimate personal care.

Nurses should recognise that human sexuality finds expression in different ways. The nurse needs to show understanding of all relationships between people and the respect to be accorded to 'the individual' and his need for confidence and privacy.

The nursing student should be aware of ways in which her own behaviour may be provocative to others — and should also recognise the influence she has on her patient and learn how to cope with sexual advances.

7   Personal cleansing and dressing

The choice of individual clothing once again has a strong cultural influence although it is also affected by the climate and fashions of the time. Good grooming is generally commended, and cleanliness is considered of great importance. In general people are considered to have a social responsibility to maintain personal cleanliness of themselves and their clothing. It is also important from the aspect of caring for the skin — an important protective organ in the body's defence system. As well as skin care, attention to hair, nails, teeth, mouth and perineal toilet are all important aspects of personal hygiene.

For most people hygiene is a personal concern which is carried out in private or in the presence of close family members. Attitude and customs associated with cleanliness have a cultural basis and nursing students should remember this, e.g. a strict observance of the Koran. For others, bathing and showering are relaxing and enjoyable and lead to a feeling of added confidence knowing that one is suitably dressed and groomed. Sometimes clothing is used as an added protection for the body, such as against rain, wind or indeed intense sunlight and more obviously in the use of crash helmets. Most people dress for personal pleasure and clothes are a means of communication.

8 Controlling body temperature

Normal body temperature in an adult is between 36°C and 37.5°C and its maintenance is important for the efficient functioning of the many chemical reactions which take place in the body. The internal mechanism which regulates the body temperature is situated in part of the hypothalamus in the brain. All metabolic processes produce heat and this is balanced by the needs at rest. However, if too much heat is produced the peripheral blood vessels dilate and heat is lost from the surface of the body. At the same time an increase in sweating occurs leading to further heat loss by evaporation. If the body temperature drops the peripheral blood vessels constrict, reducing heat loss from the body's surface. At the same time the surface hairs are raised in order to trap heat next to the body and insulate it. As most of the heat produced by the body comes from skeletal muscular activity, shivering may occur as this greatly increases additional heat.

Most people dress appropriately according to the climate in which they live as this reduces the amount of work required of the heat regulating centre. It is also possible to regulate the temperature of most homes by either warming or cooling the air.

There is a normal fluctuation in body temperature throughout the day, being slightly higher in the evening. It is also elevated by a small amount — up to 0.5°C in women during the second half of the menstrual cycle following ovulation and during the first trimester of pregnancy. An increase in exercise can cause a slight rise as a result of muscular activity, and sometimes there is a rise after a meal due to increased digestive activity.

9 Moving independently

Independent movement is of the greatest importance to all animals. In the human being it not only enables the movements from one place to another or a change in position from standing to sitting for example, but allows the individual to perform skilful tasks such as writing, speaking, smiling, engaging in eye contact, or other aspects of communication. Movement takes place by the action of skeletel muscles on the joints of the skeleton as a result of stimulation from the nervous system. The acquisition of these motor skills begins in very early childhood and continues throughout life. The human brain seems to have an infinite capacity for learning new skills. The level of achievement which can be developed with training is phenomenal (e.g. gymnastics, running a mile in less than 4 min, or playing a musical instrument). The ability to move independently is important in order to carry out many of the other activities of daily living which have been discussed. When watching an infant strive to walk the intense need for independent movement becomes clear. The elderly struggle to stay mobile as long as possible for with this mobility comes independence.

A great deal has been written recently about the importance of exercise in general health and the prevention of illness such as hypertension, coronary heart disease and obesity. This may well be associated with the fact that the expenditure of physical energy results in the relaxation of both body and mind.

10 Working and playing

The purpose of work is for earning money in order to live comfortably in a materialistic society in which success is measured by possessions and lifestyle.

The remuneration received is used to pay for a place to live which is part of the making of a safe environment, and when this is dealt with some of the remainder is usually spent on recreational activities or playing. The remainder (if there is any) may well be saved again as part of the safety need 'for a rainy day'.

The need for satisfaction from the type of employment undertaken varies among people. For some it is more important than others. However, the need for gainful employment seems to be more deep seated than was at one time realised and being unemployed appears to affect self-esteem. In the days of rising unemployment in this country considerable research is being undertaken to ascertain the attitudes of the unemployed, both those who have worked and are now redundant, and those who have left school and have never been employed.

Recreational activities are a well developed industry these days, providing employment for a large number of people. As a result they are often expensive and some leisure pursuits are financially out of reach of lower paid workers and the unemployed living on social security. However, not all activities of play are expensive and many develop hobbies which are absorbing and relatively inexpensive. Recreational activities can be relaxing or energetic, carried out alone or with a group and are very much a matter of individual choice.

11 Sleeping

Sleeping is an important activity in daily living. Without adequate sleep the degree of rest required for the repair of the body will not be achieved and the resulting fatigue will reduce the person's resources for adaptation and recovery.

There are three stages of sleep:

1. Wakefulness.
2. Synchronised sleep.
3. Desynchronised sleep.

The synchronised/desynchronised cycle takes place several times throughout a 'normal' night. Desynchronised sleep is recognised by rapid eye movement (REM) which can be seen beneath closed lids. It is less restful than the deep sleep (NREM) in which no rapid eye movements are seen. The cycle of REM and NREM sleep takes between 75 and 95 minutes, so a person sleeping for 8 hours spends 6½–7 hours in NREM/deep sleep and 1–1½ hours in REM sleep. The nurse should be aware that it takes some time to go into NREM/deep sleep and the patient needs to stay in that state for some time in order to benefit (Hernandez, 1965).

Dreams occur during sleep, although the extent to which they are recalled during waking hours will vary from person to person. The events in the dreams may be so real to an individual that he believes they have actually taken place. Some people are very frightened by dreams (nightmares) and are afraid to go to sleep for this reason.

12 Dying

This is the final stage of the activities of life which all living creatures undergo. The process of dying and the support of the patient and his family is considered to be of the greatest importance (see chapter on Care of the Dying).

The patient's admission to hospital and the planning of his care

The process of being admitted into hospital has often been a mechanical, frustrating and frightening experience for the person subjected to it.

The admission procedure is something that is taught at an early stage of nursing training. It is a procedure in which she soon becomes practised, and hopefully proficient and this can sometimes lead her to forget that admission into hospital is an important and significant event in the life of the patient and his family. When considering the number of elements which may affect a patient coming into hospital the challenge of making this a positive experience for that person, becomes significant to the success of the entire procedure. The routine procedures carried out by most hospitals may seem to be depersonalising in themselves and the warmth and understanding of the admitting nurse are of the greatest importance in mitigating the effects of this procedure.

Fact sheet 1: Planning care with an awareness of different cultural customs and needs

Mrs Khan has been admitted to a woman's surgical ward for an operation for acute appendicitis. She is Bengali, and a devout Muslim, with little understanding of English. Her husband, and her eleven year old son have accompanied her — they both understand English, and the child speaks English fluently.

Consider the following problems:

What information will the nurse require from the relatives before they leave?

How much information will she ask them to relay to Mrs Khan?

What particular problems will this patient have, on entering a women's ward?

What help can the nurse give her to overcome these?

Aspects of her nursing care which need to be considered include the following:

1. The Islamic religion as embodied by the Koran sets down rules for every aspect of life; running a family; inheritance; divorce; dress; etiquette; food; hygiene; crime and punishment; economics and business practices.
2. Trying to live and survive comfortably in the different cultural environment of Britain, yet practising her religion and preserving her own cultural identity, will pose problems for Mrs Khan.

1 Dress and hygiene

1. She must keep her body covered — especially the legs and shoulders. It may therefore be necessary to ask relatives to bring in long nightdresses for her to wear — not only in bed but also she may wish to wear it in the bath.
2. If she is unable to plait and put up her hair she will need the nurse's assistance — or the assistance of one of her relatives.
3. Nose jewels and religious medallions should not be removed unless essential for surgery or other treatment, and if this is necessary a full explanation, in simple clear words, should be given to Mrs Khan and her relatives, before her permission is given.
4. Mrs Khan will need water for washing her anal and vulval area and her hands after visiting the lavatory, using a commode or bedpan.
5. A bowl of water for hand washing will be required for Mrs Khan if she wishes to pray.
6. The left hand is considered dirty — particular difficulties will arise if this hand is immobilised.

2 Diet

Meat for Mrs Khan must be 'Halal' and pork is forbidden. Some hospitals provide deep frozen halal food. Otherwise rice, pulses and curried meat or fish is acceptable. Hot sweetened milk is a useful source of protein.

Food containing, or in contact with, forbidden ingredients will not be eaten.

The right hand is used to eat food, which is scooped off the plate with chapatis. If Mrs Khan's right hand is immobilised, she will be unable to use her left hand — which is considered dirty — and will need help with both eating and drinking.

The patient is required to wear an identity band and in many hospitals is required to get undressed and wear either his own or the hospital's night clothes. This makes him feel very vulnerable and insecure and his feeling is further intensified if relatives who may have accompanied him are requested to take his outdoor clothing home. He feels trapped and unable to escape and out of control of the situation in which he finds himself. This anxiety can be reduced by explaining the problems encountered when patients' personal property is damaged or lost, and that the hospital encourages families to keep their property in the safety of the home. However, if a patient wishes to keep his personal belongings with him he should be allowed to do so — as long as he understands his liability in the matter.

Another way of reducing anxiety during the patient's admission to hospital is to include the family as much as possible. This is especially important if the patient is disabled or is very dependent on other family members for care at home. When the patient is settled he should be introduced to other people who are in beds close to his and shown the bathroom and toilet areas as well as any other ward areas which he might like to use, such as a day or television room. He should be made aware of meal times and he and his family should have a chance to discuss visiting times or any other problems. Finally, the patient should be given time with the family member(s) who have accompanied him, and the nurse should provide as quiet a place as possible for them to say goodbye to each other. A private conversation with the family member can uncover any further problems they may foresee, and the nurse may offer reassurance and support.

When a person becomes a patient he is changing his role and with it his social identity. The company director and the man who empties dustbins look similar when in pyjamas in bed. Both have the added adjustment of handing over the control of their lives to others whose youth may provide grounds for feelings of insecurity, even though they are qualified. Whenever changes such as this are made they are accompanied by rituals which mark the event and make it clearly recognisable to all who are involved. This behaviour is called 'rites of passage' and was first described by a French anthropologist Arnold Van Gennep in 1909, when he described the rites of separation, transition and aggregation. The person who has to undergo the change has to rid himself of his previous attachments. Removing his day clothing and having his personal things taken home can be described as part of this ritual. In the transition phase the person has left his old status behind and has not yet assumed the new one. During this period he may be withdrawn and anxious. He will observe his fellow patients and the ward routine until he learns the rules and makes friends with other patients, then the aggregation phase takes place and he is accepted and accepts the new community.

An understanding of some of these concepts is of the greatest importance when the nurse considers the admission of a patient into hospital. The reaction of individuals varies enormously and must be dealt with patiently and kindly. There are few moves in life that are more ominous than the move from the home to the hospital. Thoughts may occur centring around pain and disfigurement, and even death. Very few approach an operation without fear. Individuals who are normally anxious will become more so but even relatively pragmatic individuals demonstrate some anxiety, especially if they have never been in hospital before.

Lack of privacy is noticed very quickly and also the large number of people that may be involved in the patient's care each day. The nurse is coordinator of care and should endeavour to explain the role of each of those people. When the diagnosis has not been established, the results of each test assume monumental importance and no news is usually construed by the patient as bad rather than good news. The importance of information giving was unequivocally demonstrated by Hayward (1973), in his research document.

Plan of care using the nursing process

The adjustment of the patient to hospital may affect his willingness to cooperate and accept the treatment offered. There are vast differences in both the physical and mental conditions of patients admitted to hospital and an individual plan of care needs to be made out for each of them. One approach which can be used to plan this care uses the nursing process.

The nursing process is a problem-orientated approach to planning which promotes continuous total patient care. It is centred on the person and not on his diagnosis and emphasis is placed on clear documentation. The purpose of this approach is to offer the best possible care to each patient based on his individual needs. There are four parts to the process. In the first or assessment stage the nurse talks to the patient about his illness and collects information which she can then use in the second or planning stage. The patient's problems are identified and his nursing care based on finding solutions to these problems. Aims or goals can be then expressed together with a target date and the nurse is then ready to prescribe the care necessary to achieve those aims. Nurse and patient/client are then ready to go forward together to enable the patient to achieve the optimum level of physical and mental health (or a comfortable and peaceful death). Evaluating the patient's progress and the effectiveness of the care given is a continuous process and the target and plans are updated according to their effectiveness. Whenever possible, the patient should take part in this evaluation — he is the centre to which planning and the giving of care are directed.

The assessment part of the nursing process is carried out as soon as is practical after the patient has been admitted. It should be done as soon as sufficient time is available and the interview should take place as quietly and as privately as possible. It may be appropriate to take the patient to the day room or to a quiet part of the ward. Drawing a bedside curtain is another way of producing a more personal and intimate setting and the nurse should pull up a chair and sit down beside the patient. She should always ask permission to interview the patient and might explain that she is seeking information that will make his stay in hospital more comfortable and discover any special needs that the patient might have. This is called taking a nursing history.

The completeness of the nursing history depends on the effectiveness of communication. It sets up a special working relationship between the nurse or nursing student and the patient. Many patients comment that is the first time anyone has shown such a special interest in them, and in the main they enjoy discussing their worries and anxieties with the nurse. From the nurse's point of view it is an opportunity to really get to know the new patient who has recently come into her care. She should be aware, however, that interviewing skills must be developed just in the same way as practical skills are and she should not expect to be adept at these skills at the beginning of the training.

As well as learning how to listen she must also learn how to observe her patient and notice the 'non-verbal cues' which he may give her regarding his thoughts and feelings about being in hospital. It is usually best to begin by checking that his personal details, next of kin and general practitioner are correct. This is not only a very important part of accuracy and record keeping but also sets up a rapport and the nurse can learn much about the patient and his family and socio-economic status by listening carefully to the information he is giving her. She should then begin to know what other information is relevant in order to plan the care that the patient will require while in hospital. For example, if a patient has been admitted for surgery to the hip there is no need to keep him in hospital till he can safely climb stairs if he lives in a ground floor flat. On the other hand, adequate washing facilities are desirable if a patient is possibly to undergo bowel surgery and be left with a stoma. If this facility is in any way in doubt, further questioning and discussion should take place soon after admission so that planning for discharge from hospital can take place at the very earliest opportunity, calling on whatever 'back up' facilities may be required.

Other areas to explore include whether or not the patient has been in hospital before and if so how he feels about it. He may have been very nauseated following anaesthetic on his last admission or be concerned due to the lack of pain relief. Reassurance can be given that medication is available to prevent recurrence of these situations with a considerable reduction in anxiety.

Fact sheet 2: Importance of previous experience of hospitals

The fear of losing independence is often aggravated by the memory of a previous hospital admission and a complete nursing history endeavours to highlight these areas where problems may arise, this can be clearly demonstrated anecdotally. A 46-year-old woman was admitted to the gynaecology ward. She had three children and had been admitted to the gynaecology ward for a Manchester Repair as she had stress incontinence.

Definition

Manchester Repair — anterior colporrhaphy, amputation of cervix and posterior colpoperineorrhaphy.

She had also been treated by the Rheumatology Department for rheumatoid arthritis, a condition which was well controlled at the time of her present admission. When the nurse who was admitting her talked about an earlier admission and asked about any problems or worries which arose out of it, her patient described the humiliation she had felt when she had been incontinent of urine. Further discussion revealed that the pain she experienced from her arthritis was at its worst when she woke in the morning. She had been placed some distance from the lavatories and her pain and restricted movement, together with her urgency of micturition, had made it impossible to reach them in time. The first morning she had suffered a great deal of pain and embarrassment as she left a trail of urine from her bed to the lavatory, in an effort to remain independent. Subsequently she had asked for a bedpan but this had sometimes been refused by nurses who had been instructed to encourage her to be mobile. Her solution to this was twofold. She asked her husband to bring in a supply of large size sanitary towels and rubber pants. On the mornings that her pain was less severe she used one of the sanitary towels and went to the lavatory. On the days when her pain was at its worst she gave up the unequal struggle and wet the bed.

The nurse who talked to this patient when she was admitted to the gynaecological ward discussed this problem with the senior ward staff and two solutions were planned — instructions were given for her to be woken as early as she was at home and given her analgesics; next, her bed was placed near to the lavatories so that the distance she had to walk was very short. She had no incontinence and the patient changed from the tense anxious person who was admitted to a delightful 'mum' with a sense of humour which was appreciated by all around her.

Another very important area to explore with a patient at this point is his impression and understanding of his present illness. The nurse who is taking the history must understand that the extent of the patient's awareness is unimportant in itself. Some patients will be totally aware of their condition and its implications, whereas others may know nothing at all about the disease that has brought them into hospital. In other instances, patients may totally misunderstand the nature of their illness. At this point establishing the *extent* of the patient's knowledge is the main task and this information should be shared with the other staff members. In this way each member of the team is aware of the way that the patient should be approached, using appropriate communications in the information they give. When the nurse has collected all the information she requires, she can begin to discuss with the patient the plans for his care. Involving the patients at this stage seems to establish cooperation in the future. Asking about his expectations for this admission gives guidelines for the care, and misconceptions can be dealt with at an early stage.

Finally the nurse should give the patient an opportunity to ask any questions he wants to and be sure that he is clear about the relevant logistical items he needs to know such as the ward layout, visiting times, meal times and the times he is due to have any investigations or surgery if she is aware of them. She should conclude by thanking the patient for talking to her.

(a) Writing the care plan — with the patient

The nurse is now ready to write the plan for the patient's care. The key to a successful outcome is to write the care plan from the perspective of the patient and his family. The patient is the expert about how he feels and what his needs are. However, the nurse has to produce a care plan that is accurate and realistic within the confines of the system in which she works. She should encourage the patient to take responsibility for his own problems, in so far as he is able, and the care plan should aim to support his recovery as an independent member of society.

She should begin by identifying the patient's problems and needs. Such general categories to be explored include the problems of pathology, his signs and symptoms; any emotional and spiritual difficulties which might affect his care; and social problems relating to the patient and his family, such as housing, finance, and work. Although the fundamental reason for his admission to hospital is his medical diagnosis, and hence his medical treatment which the nurse must always know and understand, the medical diagnosis is in itself rarely a nursing problem.

Nursing problems can in the main be divided into two types, usual and unusual.

1 Usual problems

These can be described as a predictable difficulty or concern experienced by many patients with the same diagnosis. These may range from post-operative pain, or fear of death prior to undergoing open heart surgery, to unconsciousness or respiratory problems following a stroke.

2 Unusual problems

These are specific to that patient at that point in time. It may be anxiety about the future if he has just been made redundant or there may be additional physiological problems. For example, the patient who has come in for the repair of an inguinal hernia may also have diabetes mellitus, or the patient for cholecystectomy may have epilepsy. Less dramatically, the elderly gentleman admitted for prostatectomy might be deaf. Planning communication is certainly made easier if this fact is taken into account, particularly if the deafness is more profound in one ear than it is in the other.

Before the care can be planned, a brief statement of the case of a problem is required. Breathlessness due to myocardial infarction would not be treated in the same way as breathlessness due to an acute exacerbation of chronic bronchitis, for example. Similarly, pain following surgery may not be treated in the same way as pain due to secondary carcinoma.

The medical diagnosis can be helpful to the nurse in anticipating and understanding her patient's problems. For example:

depression due to facial disfigurement from lacerations;
incontinence due to urinary tract infection;
incontinence due to unconsciousness.

3 Potential problems

Much of the work that nurses actually do involves trying to prevent problems from arising, and nursing skills involve recognising patients that are at a high risk. This has resulted in the development of a category for potential problems so that the appropriate nursing care can be planned and documented. For example:

skin breakdown due to immobility as a result of multiple sclerosis;
post-operative haemorrhage due to haemophillia;
skin breakdown due to age (78 years) and poor nutritional state.

Using this knowledge a selection of problems unique to each patient can be identified and aims or goals set to overcome or prevent further difficulty.

When carrying out this part of the planning, the nurse should have three main thoughts in mind.

1. The aims she is setting should be measurable so that she can evaluate their effectiveness.

2. They should also be realistic. Aims which are totally out of reach of patient and nurse alike have the effect of slowing down progress, not accelerating it.
3. Also, aims should always have a target date at which their effectiveness should be evaluated.

This does not mean to say that the care is only evaluated on the target date. It will, of course be assessed all the time. The frequency of checking should be indicated on the care plan. It can be any time from quarter hourly to once a shift, to once a week or even longer, as may be the case in psychiatry for example.

These points can be clarified by using examples:

Example 1

Problem	Aim	Frequency	Target
6th April: Pain in back and right leg due to secondary carcinoma	1. Patient quiet and relaxed in bed		7th April
	2. States that pain is absent or has decreased	2 hourly	

So in this case the patient should be questioned about his pain 2 hourly and the effectiveness of the treatment assessed after 24 hours. If the pain is absent or has decreased the nurse may decide that the treatment should be continued and a new target date set, perhaps the following day. However, if there has been no improvement in the problem, she may feel that another form of treatment is indicated, and will discuss this with the doctor.

(b) Team work

Although emphasis has been put upon nursing problems and nursing care, even greater emphasis should be placed on the team work involved in caring for the patient. The role of the nurse is central to this team. She spends more time with the patients than any of the other members — medical staff, physiotherapists, occupational therapists, speech therapists — and should develop the role of advocate representing the patient's interests to them all. In the example of the patient in pain, the nurse should report that the pain is not controlled and ask for a change or increase in medication.

Categories which can be used when stating aims include statements by patients such as 'I have no pain', or 'I feel more confident about going home'. An improvement in physical condition can also be used, for example, temperature less than 38°C or urinary output at least 1.5 litres a day. Alternatively, a descriptive phrase about the patient's behaviour can be used such as 'able to transfer safely from bed to wheelchair unaided' or 'able to walk from bed to dayroom using Zimmer frame', or 'can walk up two flights of stairs without getting breathless'.

The evaluation of care is done using the nursing progress notes. (The writer feels strongly that evaluation should not take place on the care plans.) The frequency of checking gives guidelines about what should be included and how often. Examples of the use of care plans set out in this way follow. As can be seen they are really very versatile.

Example 2: Mr Brian English

Mr Brian English is a 45-year-old executive in an insurance firm. He is married with two children of 13 and 15 years old and lives 30 miles out of central London where he works. At an important and rather stormy board meeting one day he noticed he had some pain in his chest but it lasted for a short time only and he soon forgot about it. The meeting ran late and he was hurrying to catch his train when the pain returned, it was severe and he felt like a crushing band around his chest and it was difficult for him to breathe. He doubled over and leant against a wall. A passer-by asked him if he was all right and he straightened to reassure her. The next thing he remembers is lying on the pavement. The woman was telling him that someone had called an ambulance.

Mr English was brought into the accident and emergency department where he had a chest X-ray, and an ECG confirmed the diagnosis of myocardial infarction. An intravenous infusion was set up and he was transferred to the coronary care unit for observation and monitoring of his heart beat. He was worried about his wife who had been contacted by the nursing staff in the

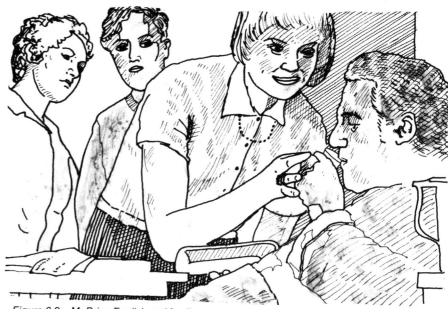

Figure 6.2   Mr Brian English and family

emergency and accident department and was on her way to the hospital. He also had some important papers in his brief case which would be needed at his office the following day. The nursing care plan is shown in Table 6.1.

Table 6.1   Nursing care plan for Mr Brian English

Date	Problem	Aim	Nursing care	Frequency	Target date
1.8	1. Pain due to myocardial infarction	Patient resting peacefully and says he's pain free	Given 1/M Diamorphine and monitor progress	Immediately check 2 hourly	
1.8	2. Anxiety due to: (a) Emergency admission (b) Diagnosis (c) Effect on family (d) Papers in brief case	Reduce anxiety to a minimum by discussing and dealing with problems systematically	1. Explain purpose of monitoring electrodes 2. Offer to discuss situation with patient and wife when she arrives 3. Organise telephone call to his office in morning to have someone come and get papers		Tomorrow a.m.
1.8	3. Possibility of cardiac arrythmia due to abnormal electrical activity from damaged tissue 4. Further damage	Reduce likelihood to minimum, observe and report abnormalities as soon as they arise Keep patient rested and quiet	1. Measure and record pulse 2. Measure and record B/P 3. Observe ECG recording — record strip 4. Sit upright in bed 5. Give oxygen using M.C. mask (high %) 6. Ensure requirements are within reach	½ hourly ½ hourly 1 hourly maintain	2.8
1.8	Possibility of collapse due to circulatory failure	Reduce demands on heart. Be prepared to act quickly should this occur Maintain a slow intravenous infusion for drug administration if needed	1. Patient should be kept resting in bed and should understand reason for this 2. Measure and chart any urine passed (routine test 1st spec) 3. Careful observation and maintenance of I.v. rate		

Example 3: Mr Mark Jacobson

Mr Mark Jacobson is a 72-year-old man who has been relatively fit throughout his life. This morning, as always, he got up to make a cup of tea for his wife. She heard a crash and when she reached the kitchen she found him lying on the floor unconscious. She ran to a neighbour's flat and they helped her to get her husband into bed and telephoned for the Doctor. He said that they should phone for an emergency ambulance which they did and Mr Jacobson was taken to the Emergency and Accident Department of the local hospital. There a stroke was diagnosed and Mr Jacobson was admitted to a medical ward; his wife went with him.

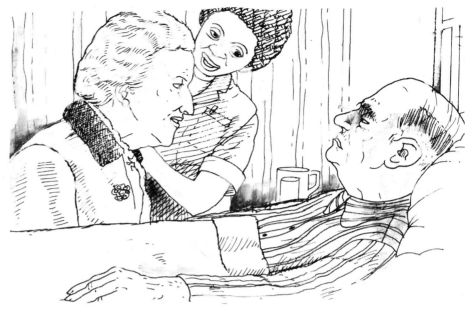

Figure 6.3   Mr Mark Jacobson and his wife

After he had been made comfortable in bed the nurse took Mrs Jacobson to see him and then sat down with her to take a nursing admission history. She told Mrs Jacobson that she could stay at the hospital if she wanted to but as her husband's condition was relatively stable she decided to go home and telephone some family and friends. Her son had already been informed of his father's illness and had arrived at the hospital to look after his mother. The nurse made sure that Mrs Jacobson knew how to contact the hospital and that the ward staff could reach her. She told her that she could visit at any time and Mrs Jacobson said she would return to the hospital in a couple of hours.

The nurse then developed a care plan at the outset (Table 6.2).

Mr Jacobson had three grown-up children who were all married with families of their own. They were a close family who rallied round immediately to support their mother. They visited their father often and during the first 48 hours of his admission there was often a family member sitting with him talking quietly. They felt that their father knew they were there.

Table 6.2   Nursing care plan for Mr Mark Jacobson

Date	Need or problem	Aim	Nursing care	Frequency	Target or review date
10.12	1. Possible respiratory complications due to unconsciousness	1. Deep regular respirations 2. Respiration rate 16–24/min 3. Temperature less than 58°C 4. Pink fingers, toes — mucous membranes	1. Position on side using Guedels airway if required and remove pharyngeal secretions by suction if necessary 2. Turn from side to side and support affected limbs, position with pillows behind back and between knees	1 hourly 2 hourly	Each shift Each shift
10.12	2. Change in neurological status following stroke	1. Stable neurological status within normal limits for patient 2. No new evidence of deficit	1. Establish and record baseline values for neurological observations 2. Measure and record neurological observations (report changes to senior nurse) 3. Talk to patient every time you approach him to carry out his care. Explain each function	Once on admission ½ hourly Always	Each shift
10.12	3. Poor nutrition and fluid intake as unconscious	1. Urine output not less than 1.2 litres/day 2. Fluid intake not less than 1.5 litres/day 3. Weight loss not more than 1.5 kg/week	1. Pass nasogastric tube and give feeds following turns, 250 ml 2. Maintain an accurate fluid intake and output chart 3. Weigh twice a week	2 hourly Daily Tues and Fri	11.12 17.12 17.12

Table 6.2 Nursing care plan for Mr Mark Jacobson — contd.

Date	Need or problem	Aims	Nursing care	Frequency	Target or review date
10.12	4. Unable to control bladder and bowels as unconscious	1. Keep clean and dry at all times 2. Avoid constipation 3. Avoid skin redness and breakdown 4. Be aware that retention of urine is a complication of this condition	1. Apply condom drainage system 2. Check and chart urine output 3. Report reduction in urine output 4. Check for skin redness and report if present 5. Chart every bowel action and report if no action for 3 days or frequent loose stools. Use barrier cream for protection of skin	2 hourly 2 hourly 2 hourly 2 hourly	Each shift
10.12	5. Unable to perform normal needs of hygiene	1. Keep clean and well groomed 2. Prevent problems associated with unconsciousness not already dealt with	1. Give bed bath 2. Clean mouth using . . . 3. Give eye care and ensure eyes closed especially prior to turning 4. Keep hair tidy when turning 5. Shave	Daily 4 hourly 4 hourly 2 hourly Daily	
12.12	6. Respiratory complications due to immobility and swallowing difficulty	1. Respiratory rate between 16 and 24/min 2. Temperature less than 38°C	1. Change position 2. Encourage coughing Work with physiotherapist 3. Take and record temperature	2 hourly 4 x daily	15.12

During the first 48 hours there was little change in his overall condition which remained stable. Then he began to be more responsive and it was clear that he recognised family members. As yet he hadn't spoken but seemed to be trying to.

Throughout the next three weeks, Mr Jacobson made good steady progress and his care plan was modified accordingly (Table 6.3).

Table 6.3 Modified care plan for Mr Jacobson

Date	Need or problem	Aims	Nursing care	Frequency	Target or review date
12.12	7. Poor nutrition and fluid intake due to swallowing difficulty	Aims as before	Give additional drinks of 200 ml Help to eat meals and clean mouth afterwards Find out favourite foods and ask family to bring in Continue to keep fluid balance chart Weigh twice a week	2 hourly Daily Tues and Fri	18.12
12.12	8. Some loss of control with bladder and bowels	Maintain continence. Avoid constipation	Take to lavatory or give urinal, encourage mobility. Report if 3 days with no bowel action. Give extra fruit and vegetables in diet, and bran	2 hourly	18.12
13.12	9. Difficulty with activities of daily living: hygiene; eating and drinking; moving about; communicating	1. Can maximise functional reserves and safely participate in as many activities as possible 2. Can make needs known	1. Give bed bath or aid with bathing according to patient's wishes 2. Aid with eating and drinking independently by using non-slip mat under plate, cutting up food or using a plate guard. Place a drink within reach of patient 3. Praise all independent activity 4. Speak slowly and directly using short sentences, give him time to reply. Talk to speech therapist and reinforce her work 5. Help out of bed into a chair twice a day for meals	Daily Mealtimes Always Always Always 11–1300 hours	18.12 20.12 20.12 20.12 18.12

Table 6.3   Modified care plan for Mr Jacobson

Date	Need or problem	Aims	Nursing care	Frequency	Target or review date
16.12			6. Help to walk to day room for meals using zimmer frame	17–1900 hours	
20.12	10. Depression due to frustration with limitations and fear about the future and changes in social status	1. Can express fears and anxieties to family and nurse 2. Has realistic expectations of his own ability	1. Talk to patient and suggest ways he can handle his difficulties	Often	
			2. Make sure he is clear about the use of the equipment he is using, e.g. walking frame	Daily	
			3. Discuss progress and find out how he would like to be supported when discharged		28.12
			4. Involve family with care as much as possible, e.g. meals, speech therapy, bathing, walking	Always	
	11. Need for discharge teaching	1. Patient and family express understanding of limitation of lifestyle and of medical treatment	11. Encourage family to become more involved with patient care 2. Work with physiotherapist and occupational therapist to achieve continuity of care 3. Encourage patient and family to express fears about discharge and help them to resolve them together 4. Ensure Mrs Jacobson understands medication		
30.12			5. Liaise with district nurse and organise visit at home following discharge		Discharged 31.12.82.

Example 4: Mrs Evelyn Jones

Mrs Evelyn Jones is 45 years old and has worked in a large department store for 15 years since her youngest child was able to go to school. At first she worked part time but for the last 10 years has worked full time and is now the supervisor for her area. As a young woman Mrs Jones was troubled by varicose veins which became worse during her two pregnancies. She had them injected following the birth of her second child with some improvement at the time, but over the last five years they had become much worse. They not only looked tortuous and unsightly but caused Mrs Jones some pain and swelling by the end of the day.

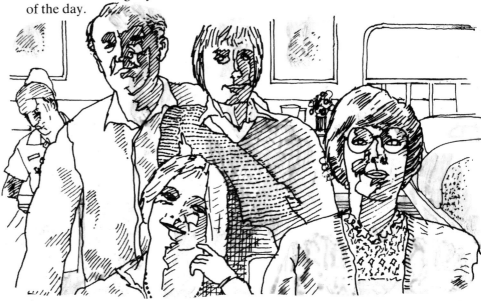

Figure 6.4   Mrs Evelyn Jones and family

Table 6.4   Nursing care plan for Mrs Evelyn Jones

Date	Need or problem	Aims	Nursing Care
12.12	Needs to be prepared for surgery	1. Understands surgery and anaesthetic 2. Appreciates need for physical preparation 3. Knows what to expect post-operatively	1. Check patient understands doctor's explanation of operation and supplement it if necessary 2. Give opportunity to express anxiety if she has any 3. Explain need for leg and pubic shaves prior to carrying these out 4. Give two glycerine suppositories as bowels not open today 5. Explain that she should not eat or drink anything after breakfast tomorrow — surgery 1500 hours 6. Make sure doctor has prescribed pre-medication and post-operative analgesia 7. Explain that she will experience some discomfort post-operatively and that analgesics will be available and she should ask for them 8. Ask physiotherapist to visit Monday a.m. as patient smokes 20–30 cigarettes a day
	Operation Bilateral stripping and ligation of varicose veins Returned to ward 16.40 hours 13.12.82		

Nursing care plan for Mrs Evelyn Jones (post-operatively)

Date	Need or problem	Aim	Nursing care	Frequency	Target or review date
13.12	Possible complications following surgery	1. Prevention of same 2. Patient expresses that she is comfortable and pain free	1. Sit up and encourage to cough. Give sputum pot	When awake	14.12
			2. Enquire about post-operative pain, give analgesic if required	4 hourly	14.12
			3. Encourage leg and foot movement in conjunction with physiotherapist	1 hourly	14.12
			4. Examine wound sites for oozing, keep dry at all times	1 hourly	14.12
			5. Make sure bandages remain intact	1 hourly	14.12
			6. Allow to drink small amounts. Watch for post anaesthetic nausea. Inform senior nurse if this occurs	When she asks	14.12
			7. Wash face and hands and change into own nightdress. Brush hair	Before husband visits	14.12
			8. Settle comfortably for night. Explain need for her to sit up following anaesthetic	At night	14.12
			9. Observe throughout the night	1 hourly	14.12
14.12	Needs to mobilise	1. Prevention of complications of surgery 2. Patient aware of her part in this	1. Continue to encourage deep breathing and coughing	2 hourly	18.12
			2. Change sputum pot and examine for possible infection	Daily 6 a.m.	18.12
			3. Discourage from smoking		
			4. Teach to apply own bandages	a.m.	
			5. Explain that she should not sit in chair but may sit on bed with legs straight and should walk about for five minutes in every hour	a.m.	
			6. Strip and spray wounds	a.m.	16.12
15.12	Prepare for discharge		1. Arrange date for Mrs Jones to come to hospital for removal of sutures		
			2. Liaise with doctor for analgesic. Arrange out-patient appointment for 6/52		
			3. Arrange for patient's family to come and collect her		Discharged 16.12.82

She had been referred for hospital consultation some two years previously and her name was put on the waiting list for surgery. On two previous occasions she had received an admission letter but on both her admissions had been deferred at the last minute due to the admission of an emergency. Finally she arrived in the women's surgical ward on Sunday afternoon for surgery the following day. After she had been shown to her bed and sorted out her belongings with her family they went home leaving her feeling rather lonely and unsure of herself but none the less glad to be having her surgery at long last.

A nurse came along to take a nursing admission history and following this she developed a nursing care plan (Table 6.4) to cover the period up to Mrs Jones's surgery the following day. Additions to the care plan were made post-operatively.

Activity

Jennifer Martin is 50 years old and is severely handicapped by multiple sclerosis. She is unable to move her legs and her left arm, and her right arm is ataxic. She has a urinary catheter permanently in position as without it she has retention of urine. This has led to repeated urinary tract infections which although treated by her GP have developed into pyelonephritis and Mrs Martin has come into hospital for investigations and treatment for this.

Although the diagnosis of multiple sclerosis was made when she was only 25, Mrs Martin has struggled hard with her disability and deterioration had thankfully been slow. Her husband and two children had supported her and she managed well at home. She had a number of household aids and was visited regularly by the GP, District Nurse and other social services. She really disliked being away from her family in hospital and wanted to go home as soon as possible.

This was her sixth hospital admission. On the previous occasion when she had influenza which had developed into pneumonia she was in for 3½ weeks and developed a pressure sore, so she felt very anxious about this admission.

Suggest a possible plan of care for Mrs Martin on this admission.

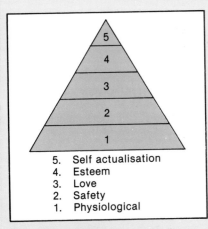

5. Self actualisation
4. Esteem
3. Love
2. Safety
1. Physiological

Figure 6.5   Maslow's theory of the hierarchy of needs

Fact sheet 3: Abraham Maslow's theory of the hierarchy of needs

Abraham Maslow developed a theory of the hierarchy of needs which is a useful way of approaching and assessing the patient's needs and activities of daily living. He describes five levels of need — sometimes expressed as a pyramid in diagram (Figure 6.5).

These needs develop in turn from the basic level as the child grows up, the physical needs remaining below the level of consciousness as long as they are reasonably satisfied for the individual. Each higher need appears only when these lower levels are met to the individual's satisfaction. In conditions of deprivation, however, they emerge and dominate the behaviour of the person. Dominant needs tend to become increasingly dominant, absorbing more and more of the individual's attention (Vernon, 1969).

(a) Physiological needs

This need comprises all the needs for oxygen, food and water as well as the salts and vitamins required for normal homeostasis in the body. Elimination would also be included in this group of needs together with the maintenance of a comfortable environment and body temperature. It is perhaps a paradox that these are the strongest needs — as the average person will not give much thought to where his next molecules of oxygen, salt or water are coming from. Maslow says that these needs must be satisfied before the next ones can be met. When these needs are not met for any period of time survival itself is threatened and satisfaction of deprived needs takes precedence over all else.

The nurse must never underestimate the importance of these basic needs. The breathless patient is fighting for his life and is only interested in this. Although malnutrition is not seen frequently in the Western World the vagrant or the elderly may well be undernourished and more interested in food than anything else when first admitted to hospital. The nurse should also remember the basic nature of the need for food and water when they are withdrawn as part of a patient's treatment. An adequate explanation of how that need will be met throughout the period of starvation is of the greatest importance and can reduce anxiety enormously.

Many patients become pre-occupied with their bowels when they are ill and when elimination is seen as a fundamental need this pre-occupation is easily explained and the nurse's role in ensuring adequate elimination assumes a new importance. This problem arises particularly with immobile patients, and an example of how re-establishing an adequate pattern of elimination can transform the quality of a patient's life can be read in Richard Lammerton's article 'Resurrected by an Enema' (1976).

The human infant is also trained to control elimination from an early age and a great deal of importance is attached to this control. As well as this the private nature of these bodily processes is emphasised. The use of bedpans and commodes is frequently a source of embarrassment to a patient. The task of assisting patients with these needs should always be carried out with tact and the maximum amount of privacy which can be afforded him. Failure to control bladder and bowels should always be dealt with compassionately and with tact and diplomacy and the patient should be given the opportunity to talk about his incontinence and how he feels about it.

Lastly in this category comes the need for sexual expression. Maslow uses this term in its physiological sense associated with the species propagation. Sexual gratification as such is not usually high on a patient's hierarchy of need when he is seriously ill. However, the importance of sexuality should not be underestimated, particularly when an individual is unable to carry out sexual functions normally. There is increasing awareness of the sexual problems of disabled people and organisations have been formed to give support to people with disability.

There is a broader aspect which is often not given enough consideration by professional personnel. Generally we are brought up to consider a sexual relationship as an expression of love and affection between two people who are attracted to one another. Feeling attractive is closely associated with the image we have of ourselves and a change in that self-image can sometimes cause severe problems regarding sexuality. Probably the most obvious examples arise from mutilating surgery such as the removal of the breast (mastectomy). Giving the woman opportunities to express her feelings together with her partner is of the greatest importance. Other patients who experience difficulty are those with severe burns, scarring and those with generalised skin lesions. The nurse needs to be aware that these patients may consider themselves to be unattractive, so that her understanding and support can be offered.

Another group of patients who should be considered here are those who have had amputations, particularly those in the younger age groups. Lastly a problem with sexuality is usually experienced by those people undergoing bowel surgery resulting in the formation of an ileostomy or colostomy. This is an area in which much development has taken place recently leading to support groups of fellow sufferers who have experience in managing the problems which arise and who visit and support those for whom these problems are new.

Finally it must be said that for many patients admission to hospital means that their regular and satisfactory sexual relationship with their spouse must cease for a period of time. Most patients manage to cope with this situation but the nurse should be aware that it can be a stressful time and may bring worries to the surface which have hitherto been repressed. All this is not to suggest that the nurse should be a sex-counsellor but simply that she should be aware of the problems which may arise in some of these situations.

(b) Need for personal safety and a safe environment

This need is felt when physiological needs are met to the individual's satisfaction. The need for somewhere to live, sufficient money to buy requirements for physical security and possible saving for the future are examples of this need and it varies from person to person and from one social group to another. In addition, health and safety at work problems are frequently under consideration and the prevention of unsafe practices is heavily emphasised.

Generally we do not give much attention to personal safety and security except in times of emergency or periods of disorganisation of the social structure such as in times of rioting or civil war. Natural disasters such as floods or earthquake also affect our safety needs. However, many of the precautions taken to maintain safety are dependent on a secure income so during times of inflation and high unemployment these needs are more apparent in the adult population, particularly the self-employed.

The nurse may feel that her personal safety is threatened by aggressive behaviour from patients or abusive language from relatives.

At an emotional level security is often established within the family unit and therefore, removing a person from such a safe environment and admitting him into hospital will give rise to feelings of insecurity.

(c) Needs for love, affection and to belong

When the physiological and safety needs are satisfied the next class of needs in the hierarchy can be met. This need for love, affection and belonging is not supported by scientific evidence, though it can be seen in individual behaviour. It is hard to translate this into the terms of a patient in hospital. However, a warm response from the nurse, full of interest and encouragement, will certainly go a long way towards making a patient 'feel at home'. In order to help him settle and feel that he 'belongs' he must be given sufficient information about the ward layout and general day to day running such as meal times and visiting times so that the patient can begin to cope with his change of surroundings.

(d) Needs for esteem

These needs involve both self-esteem and the esteem a person receives from others. Everyone in our society has a need for a stable, firmly based high level of self-respect and respect from others. There are two components of this need. The first involves personal competence with the confidence which accompanies it, the second involves the need for acknowledgement and recognition from others. When these needs are met the person feels self-confident and valuable in the family and in society. When they are frustrated the person feels insecure and inferior, doubting his own worth.

When an individual is admitted to hospital he is removed from home and work, the two areas which provide much of the basis of his feeling competent, confident and valued. It is necessary then that the nurse appreciates the worth of every patient within her care and that all her patients have a sense of their own importance and individuality.

(e) The need for self-actualisation

According to Maslow's theory this need is activated when all the foregoing needs are achieved. He has described this state as the individual doing what he is born to do. The need makes itself felt in the form of restlessness and a feeling that something is lacking, even though the person is a secure and respected member of society. A self-actualising person has a core of characteristics. Such a person is more spontaneous than other people, has a greater acceptance of himself and others and greater perception.

This enables him to see more effectively what is actually there, rather than what it is feared may be there, and this enables acceptance and spontaneity.

World War II had a considerable effect on Abraham Maslow. It led him to consider why it is that psychology is unable to contribute anything towards world peace or to the eradication of the problems of world hunger. More about his work can be found in some of his better known books: *Motivation and Personality* (1954 and 1970), *Religious Values and Real Experiences* (1964 and 1970), *The Further Reaches of Human Nature* (completed in 1970 just before his death and published posthumously by his wife Bertha in 1971).

References

Calista, S., Riehl, R., Calista, J. P. and Calista, R. S., *Conceptual Models for Nursing Practice,* Appleton-Century-Crofts, 1974

Hayward, J., *Information — a Prescription against Pain?,* RCN, 1973

Henderson, V., *Basic Principles of Nursing Care,* ICN, 1969

Hernandez, P. R., Attention, sleep behaviour, *A Mapping of an Inhibitory System in the Brain,* National Institute of Mental Health Research Project Summaries No. 2, U.S. Govt. Printing Office, pp. 141, 143–144, 1965

Lammerton, R., Resurrected by an enema, *Nursing Times,* 21 Oct., 1976

Masters, W. H. and Johnson, V. E., *Human Sexual Response,* Little Brown and Co., 1966

Roper, N., Logan, W. and Tierney, A., *The Elements of Nursing,* Churchill Livingstone, 1980

Vernon, M. D., *Human Motivation,* Cambridge University Press, 1969

Yura, H. and Walsh, M. B., *The Nursing Process,* Appleton-Century-Crofts, 1978

Further reading

Argyle, M., *The Psychology of Interpersonal Behaviour,* Pelican, 1970

Barnett, D. E., Planning Patient Care, 1 and 2, *Nursing Times,* 1982

Cartwright, D. S., *Theories and Modes of Personality,* William C. Brown, 1978

Elhart, D. F., Cragg, S. H. and Rees, O.M., *Scientific Principles in Nursing,* 8th edn, C. V. Mosby, 1978

Henderson, V. and Nite, G., *Principles and Practice of Nursing,* 6th edn, Macmillan Inc, New York, 1978

Little, D. E. and Carnevali, D. L., *Nursing Care Planning,* 2nd edn, Lippincott 1976

Mayer, M. G., *A Systematic Approach to Nursing Care,* 2nd edn, Appleton-Century-Crofts, 1978

Miller, J., *The Body in Question,* Cape, 1978

Roper, N., Logan, W. W. and Tierney, A.J., *Learning to Use the Process of Nursing,* Churchill Livingstone, 1981

Wilson-Barnett, J., *Stress in Hospital,* Churchill Livingstone, 1979

Wu, R., *Behaviour and Illness,* Prentice-Hall, 1973

Yura, H. and Walsh, M. B., *Human Needs and the Nursing Process,* Appleton-Century-Crofts, 1978

Chapter 7

Understanding nursing research

by Jill Macleod-Clark

> 'To speculate without facts is to attempt to enter a house of which one has not the key, by wandering aimlessly round and round, searching for the walls and now and then peering through the windows. Facts are the key.'
>
> Julian Huxley *Essays in Popular Science*

Introduction

One of the most exciting changes which has occurred in nursing in recent years is the growing awareness of the importance of facts in nursing rather than a reliance upon speculation or dogma. This awareness has brought with it a growth in research activity and research knowledge, which should affect every nurse and, potentially, every aspect of nursing practice.

There is a fundamental link between standards of care and the role of research in the profession. Research is necessary in order to identify areas where improvements are needed and in order to monitor and evaluate every aspect of nursing practice. Now this does not mean that all nurses will end up being full time researchers but simply that all nurses must be 'research-minded' and understand the place of research in nursing. The Briggs Report (1972) pinpointed the need to foster research-mindedness during the nurse training and the RCN (1982) has emphasised the need to help nurses learn about research, defining 'research mindedness' as a 'critical', questioning approach to one's work, the desire and ability to find out about the latest research in that area and the ability to assess its value to the situation and apply it as appropriate' (RCN, 1982).

What is research?

Research is often seen as something very complex and mysterious, but, while it may indeed be a complex activity, it is certainly not mysterious. Indeed, quite the opposite is true, for the process of research involves an attempt to increase knowledge and discover new facts through *systematic scientific enquiry,* and any activity which is systematic cannot also be mysterious.

When research is carried out appropriately, the process can seem to be laborious and time consuming. Many people may question the value of such a process especially when guesswork, a hunch or commonsense may result in similar findings to those of a lengthy research project. The problem with commonsense ideas or hunches is that they are *subjective* — they are determined solely by the individual's opinion, attitudes or experience which may or may not be accurate. Research on the other hand gives us the tools to develop our knowledge base in a systematic and objective way. The objectivity of the research process is crucial precisely because it eliminates the bias of individual's views and attitudes. Assuming that the research has been conducted appropriately the findings carry out much more weight.

Research in nursing will result in an increase in scientifically based knowledge, but such knowledge will not always be 'new'. As has been said before, one outcome of successful research will be evidence which supports existing beliefs or practice. When this happens, people are often tempted to question the point of doing the research in the first place if all it does is confirm what was already 'known'. However, there is a world of difference between thinking or believing something and knowing something for certain, and it is this knowledge or 'the facts' which are crucial to research and to nursing.

Some research projects, or course, *will* generate completely new facts or data and, in doing so, may refute or contradict previously held beliefs, intuitions or dogma. Again such findings can prove difficult to accept because well-established habits and behaviour may have to be changed. However, whatever the results of a project, there is one almost inevitable outcome of research activity. **The systematic analysis of any problem will mean that further new questions are raised, new insights gained and new ideas generated, and these in turn all contribute to the development of new knowledge.**

How is research done?

There are many different types and scales of research activity involving a variety of research methods. However, the underlying principles of research remain similar and the steps of the research process follow a logical sequence. The main steps are:

(a) The identification of a researchable problem;
(b) a critical analysis of the existing literature in that area;
(c) designing the research project and developing the data collection instruments;
(d) assessing the feasibility of the study;
(e) data collection;
(f) analysis and interpretation of data or findings;
(g) the preparation of a research report and dissemination of findings.

A detailed description of these steps can be found in many research textbooks, some of which are listed at the end of the chapter, but each is discussed very briefly below. It is important to remember, however, that these steps are not completely separate entities. Each of them overlaps and influences other stages of the process.

(a) Identification of a researchable problem

This first step in the research process is, in many ways, the most crucial. It has often been said that quality of a research project is determined by the quality of the research question posed. It is certainly true that identifying a researchable problem and defining and refining this into appropriate research questions requires skill and experience. However, it is also a part of research which is open to all nurses, not just those actually doing 'research'. Many excellent research questions or problem areas have been generated outside the confines of a research project. Most nurses have asked themselves questions about their work — **why** they are doing a certain procedure or **why** they are using a certain technique or substance. For example, you might ask why pressure sores in one ward are treated with egg-white and oxygen while in another they are left alonbe. Or you might ask why the dressing trolley in one ward is cleaned with surgical spirit, yet in another they use soap and water.

Now in these instances, the treatment of pressure sores and the cleaning of trolleys are the identified researchable problems. From these areas many, many research questions can be generated — for example 'which is the best substance for cleaning dressing trolleys?' or even more specific, 'which is more effective, surgical spirit or soap and water?' A research question must be unambiguous and all terms must be clearly defined. For example the meaning of the word *effectively* in this context must be carefully defined and described.

(b) A critical analysis of the literature

Once the researcher's area of interest has been defined it is essential that the relevant literature in that area is located and reviewed. This stage in the research process is obviously time-consuming and demanding and it is essential that the task is approached in a systematic way. Library facilities do vary considerably from place to place but, in principle it should be possible to find one local librarian (often in a postgraduate centre, polytechnic, university or school of nursing) who will be able to help in the literature search. There is also a network of national library resources which have a special interest in nursing literature (see Macleod-Clark and Stodulski, 1978).

At the start of a literature search, the researcher may have several ideas about the subject and the eventual research question often does not emerge until the literature has been reviewed. It may be that someone has already carried out a similar project, or that the findings from other research in the area leads the researcher to think about the problem in a new way. Certainly at the end of a successful literature review the researcher should have an accurate picture of the work which has been done and should be able to focus down on a particular area. However, it is important to emphasise that reading and reviewing the literature should not be an activity which is exclusive to researchers. This is a part of the research process which can be shared by all nurses who have a professional interest in their work. Good nursing practice should be based on knowledge developed through other's research and every nurse should have a curiosity about research and an ability to track down literature in their area of interest.

(c) Designing the research project

As has been said before, the steps of the research process overlap and the researcher will have been thinking about possible research designs right from the start of the project. However, at this point a definite decision and plan will have to be made about the format to be used for the systematic collection of data. The type of design chosen will, of course, depend upon the research question or problem to be examined and may be influenced by previous work in the area.

At the broadest level research can be described as either empirical or non-empirical. In empirical research data are gathered from the 'real' work while non-empirical research does not necessarily require the collection of new data, but involves taking a philosophical, historical or theoretical approach to a problem. There are examples of such research in nursing, although they tend to be in a minority (see Schrock, 1977; White, 1978; Inman, 1975).

Examples of empirical research are more common and there are many different ways of classifying such research. Perhaps the simplest, though imperfect, classification, is the distinction between survey, experimental and descriptive research. A survey approach is usually chosen when information is required about or from large numbers of people. This information is generally collected by questionnaire or interview. The larger the sample and more representative this is, then the more appropriate it becomes to extrapolate the findings to the population as a whole. The findings from small scale surveys should not be generalised, although if the study was replicated in a different area, then similar findings may well emerge. Large scale studies although potentially very valuable are very demanding in terms of resources and for this reason, many in nursing research have been on a relatively small scale. Some larger scale surveys have been carried out (Hockey, 1972) but readers should always assess the size and representativeness of the sample used before generalising the findings.

Experimental research designs are used when the researcher is trying to measure the effect of a specific input (e.g. new treatment, drug, etc.). The design is based on the principle of using groups of subjects (experimental and control groups) which are as similar as possible in all respects except that of the input to be studied. So, for example, if the effect of a drug was being studied the experimental group would be as similar as possible to the control group in respect of age, sex, diagnosis and treatment, etc., except that the experimental group would receive the drug and the control group would not. In a properly designed experiment, any changes observed or measured in the experimental group which did not occur in the control group, could be attributed to the effect of the drug. Some experimental research has been carried out in nursing, notably studies which have tried to measure the effect of specific nursing interventions (Wilson-Barnett, 1978; Hayward, 1975; Boore, 1978).

Descriptive research designs are those which, as the label implies, set out to describe specific events, groups or individuals. There is a sense in which all research involves some description but a few studies are mostly or wholly descriptive. These can also vary in scale, though as events usually have to be observed and catalogued, very large descriptive studies are more rare. Descriptive research often takes the form of a case study where the researcher looks in depth at a small number of subjects or a limited number of events. There are many examples of descriptive research in nursing (see Hunt, 1974; Towell, 1975; Faulkner, 1980; Macleod-Clark, 1981). Such studies attempt to present an objective description of different aspects of nursing which, in turn, can be used as a basis for further research.

The above discussion of research design is, obviously, highly simplified and very superficial. For a fuller description of the area, readers are referred to the suggested booklist at the end of the chapter.

(d) Assessing the feasibility of the proposed study

This next stage in the research process is often underemphasised, but again can make all the difference between success and failure.

Feasibility must be assessed in terms of the scale of the project. Can one person cope with the work? Is there enough time? Is there enough money? It is also essential to establish whether available resources in terms of literature, expertise and commitment are adequate. Access to the appropriate area (e.g. ward, hospital, school of nursing) where data will be collected must be negotiated. Most importantly, the ethics of the proposed research must be assessed (see RCN, 1977) and every effort has to be made to ensure that the project does not involve unnecessary risks or inconvenience to patients or staff, that privacy is not invaded and that respect for confidentiality and anonymity is upheld. Wherever appropriate, ethical approval should be sought and obtained and the informed consent of all those participating in the study must always be sought.

All research should be preceded by some exploratory work which gives insight into the feasibility of the project and the reality of the problem. At this stage preliminary plans in terms of the design of the study and the methods to be used should be explored. Subsequently the actual methods chosen will be tried out (piloted) and any necessary changes made before the main data collection takes place.

(e) Data collection

The method (or methods) chosen for the collection of data in a study will again be determined by the research questions being asked. The main methods of collecting data are by observation, questioning and measurement, and some or all of these methods are often used in combination.

Observation is sometimes seen as a 'soft' option in research, but nothing could be further from the truth. One of the greatest difficulties is eliminating subjectivity or bias from the observation process. Observers have to be trained to observe as objectively and reliably as possible. When possible, two or more observers can be used to check reliability, and, increasingly, the use of audio and video equipment allow a permanent record of events to be observed which can then be analysed retrospectively. The extent to which the observer is integrated into the situation being studied can also vary. Some researchers choose to be 'participant observers' and work as part of the team they are observing (Towell, 1975). Others, more commonly, act as 'non-participant observers', trying to take no part in the activities being studied (Lelean, 1973; Hawthorn, 1974).

It is very common to find questionnaires being used as a data collection tool. These too vary in complexity and scale and can be administered during an interview by the researchers, or filled out completely independently by the subjects, then returned to the researcher. Some may even be sent by post (Cartwright, 1964). Questionnaires also vary in terms of the extent to which they are structured — some asking very tightly worded questions requiring simple yes/no answers and others asking for open-ended unstructured and fuller responses from the respondents.

Some research designs involve the use of measurement in data collection. Such measurement can be in pencil and paper form as in, for example, the assessment of anxiety (Wilson-Barnett, 1978), or in physiological form such as the measurement of stress levels determined by 17-hydrooxycorticosteroids in urine (Boore, 1978). However, whatever method of data collection is used, it goes without saying that the most important criteria of success are accuracy and objectivity. These are not easy criteria to meet and for a fuller discussion of the complexities of data collection readers are again referred to the suggested reading list at the end of the chapter.

(f) Analysis and interpretation of data or findings

Data which emerge from a study may be quantitative (i.e. they are quantifiable) or qualitative (i.e. they are descriptive and not necessarily amenable to quantification). The main principle underlying all data analysis is that it should be organised and systematic and should obviously relate to the questions asked. Not all data analysis involves 'number crunching' and not all data which are amenable to quantification require statistical analysis. On the contrary, there are many examples where statistical analysis would be quite inappropriate, especially where sample sizes are small and/or unrepresentative.

Research findings are always valuable, even if they are negative — that is, even if they do not demonstrate a hoped for relationship. What is most important is that any interpretation of the data is valid and that findings from small studies are not used to extrapolate to the world at large. All research reports should be scrutinised carefully in order to gain a clear picture of the size of the sample and the way that the data were collected before making any generalisations.

(g) Research reports and dissemination of findings

It is the researcher's responsibility to produce a report of any research undertaken and to make efforts to ensure that findings are disseminated. It is, on the other hand, every nurse's responsibility to make efforts to read such reports and seek out relevant findings. While some researchers do fail in their responsibility to disseminate findings, **it is also true that many nurses do not regularly keep up to date with nursing journals and literature. Even if they never get involved with undertaking a research project every nurse should be involved in the first and last steps in the research process. From the first day as a student nurse, until retirement day, nurses have a professional responsibility to think critically and constructively about all aspects of nursing and to keep up to date with the new knowledge generated through research findings.**

How has research influenced nursing to date?

There has been a large quantity and variety of research undertaken into nursing in the UK over the past two decades. These studies have investigated many aspects of nursing practice and procedures as well as examining areas of relevance to nursing management and education (see Macleod-Clark and Hockey, 1979). Perhaps the greatest overall impact of these studies has been in terms of the growing interest and awareness of research in nursing and the way in which they have sparked off new questions and further research. The research would seem to have had less impact in relation to obvious changes in the practice. This may, in part, be understandable in view of the small scale of many such studies. What was required in these cases was replication in order to strengthen or refute the early findings but very few replication studies have been undertaken.

However, there *are* areas of research where the evidence is compelling enough and sufficient work has been undertaken to merit some changes of practice and yet change has still been very slow to take place. Examples of this would be studies relating to temperature taking (e.g. Nichols and Kucha, 1972) or pressure area care (Norton *et al.*, 1975). The reasons for this slow response are not entirely clear. There certainly seems to have been a recent acceleration in interest in research findings with many more hospitals and units anxious to participate and consider changes in practice. However, this is by no means universal and it is still common to hear research findings being rejected out of hand or disputed without adequate basis.

The reluctance to accept the place of research findings in nursing can perhaps best be understood in terms of the confusion and threat that change can cause. For decades nursing has been a hierarchical and discipline based job, where instructions were taken from doctors and dogmatic practices handed down without question. Now nursing is changing. Nurses make decisions about nursing management, education and nursing care and in order to make informed decisions, nurses are becoming more aware that they *need* research findings.

Thus the influence of research on nursing is growing much greater but this does not mean that researchers can rest on their laurels. Their audiences will become more critical and demanding, their research must become even more rigorous and their evidence even more convincing. In essence the whole of nursing practice, education and management is open to critical analysis. Many aspects of nursing care have long been taken for granted and would benefit from close scrutiny. Examples of such aspects of nursing include well practised dressing techniques and sterile procedures. Questions which could usefully be asked include: How effective or necessary are they? How sterile are they? We do not yet know how best to treat pressure sores, although a large study on this topic is currently in progress. The implementation of the 'nursing process' and the changes this brings with it are areas which should be examined. How do such changes affect patient well being, levels of staff stress, doctor–nurse relationships, etc? The list of potential research problems or areas is endless and every nurse has an important role to play in continually raising such questions.

However, it is important to remember that the world will not change over night. At the moment we are making a start but implementing new practices and changing long-standing habits inevitably causes pain and upheaval. We, as a profession, must tread softly, but not too softly and nursing students have a specially important role to play. The impetus for research must be continually fuelled by putting research-mindedness into practice. This means asking questions, trying to find the answers and refusing to be satisfied when there are no answers. This is the basis of research.

Conclusion

The idea that research-mindedness is a vital ingredient for the nursing profession is not a new one. Over 20 years ago, Professor Brotherston ably summed up the need for nurses to develop an enquiring approach to their work:

> 'Whereas the ability and opportunity to carry out research must be limited to a minority in any profession, an urgent and understanding sense of the need for research should be a part of the mental equipment of *every* member of any profession worthy of the name. Such an attitude of mind is easy enough to command, not so easy to cultivate. Research-mindedness is the opposite of prejudice, of stereotyped thinking and rule-of-thumb action; and all of us are more or less creatures of prejudice, with a preference for imitating the traditional customs of the groups in which we live and work. Now traditional customs are comfortable and necessary things in certain circumstances, but they can be dangerous limitations to the search for knowledge and the improvement of methods of applying existing knowledge.'

(Brotherston, 1960)

This chapter began with the assertion that there have been many changes in nursing in recent years. Such changes should not make us feel complacent. As nurses become more research-minded, then nursing will change even more. Some of the changes produced by research will be painful, some will be difficult but in the final analysis research will change nursing for the better. As professionals, nurses have no choice but to contribute to such changes, because in the long run they will inevitably result in improved patient care.

References

Boore, J., *A Prescription for Recovery,* RCN, 1978

Briggs Report, *Report of the Committee on Nursing,* Command 5115, HMSO, 1972

Brotherston, J., *Learning to Investigate Problems,* Report of an International Service on Research Nursing, ICN, 1960

Cartwright, A., *Human Relations and Hospital Care,* Routledge and Kegan Paul, 1964

Faulkner, A., Communication and the nurse, *Nursing Times,* **76,** 21, Occasional Paper, 1980

Hawthorn, P., *Nurse, I Want my Mummy,* RCN, 1974

Hayward, J., *Information, a Prescription against Pain,* RCN, 1975

Hockey, L., *Women in Nursing,* Hodder and Stoughton, 1972

Hunt, J., *The Teaching and Practice of Surgical Dressings in Three Hospitals,* RCN, 1974

Inman, U., *Towards a Theory of Nursing Care,* RCN, 1975

Lelean, S., *Ready for Report, Nurse,* RCN, 1973

Macleod-Clark, J. and Stodulski, A., How to find out: A guide for searching the nursing literature, *Nursing Times,* **74**(b), Occasional Paper, 1978

Macleod-Clark, J. and Hockey, L., *Research for Nursing,* HM and M, 1979

Macleod-Clark, J., Communication in nursing, *Nursing Times,* **77,** 1, 341–347, 1981

Nichols, G. and Kucha, D., Taking adult temperatures. Oral, axillary and rectal temperature determination and relationships, *Nursing Research,* **15** (4), 307–310, 1972

Norton, D., McLaren, R. and Exton-Smith, A., *An Investigation of Geriatric Nursing Problems,* Churchill Livingstone, reprinted 1975

RCN, *Ethics Related to Research in Nursing,* RCN, 1977

RCN, *Research-mindedness and Nurse Education,* RCN, 1982

Schrock, R., *An Investigation into the Principles of Health Visiting,* CETHV, 1977

Towell, D., *Understanding Psychiatric Nursing,* RCN, 1975

White, R., *Social Change and the Development of the Nursing Profession: A Study of the Poor Law Nursing Service 1848-1948,* Kimpton, 1978

Wilson-Barnett, J., Patients' emotional responses to barium X-rays, *Journal of Advanced Nursing,* **3,** 37-46, 1978

Further reading

Fox, D. J. and Lesser, U., *Readings on the Research Process in Nursing,* Appleton-Century-Crofts, 1981

Kerlinger, F., *Foundations of Behavioural Research,* Holt, Rinehart and Winston, 1973

Krauz, E. and Miller, S., *Social Research Design,* Longmans, 1974

Robson, C., *Experiment, Design and Statistics in Psychology,* Penguin Books, 1975

Scaman, C. and Verhanick, P., *Research Methods for Undergraduate Students in Nursing,* Appleton-Century-Crofts, 1981

Yeomans, K., *Introducing Statistics.* Penguin Books, 1971

Index

Pain mechanisms, theories of, 63
Pain observation chart, 71, 76–78
Pain receptors, 65
Pain suppression theory, 63
Pain therapy, 63
Pancreas, 22, 24, 46
Parasites, 45
Pathogens, 43, 44, 45, 47–48, 49, 51, 52
  bacterial, 50
  reservoir of, 47
Pathology, 21
Patient
  assessment and management of, 33
  needs of, 53, 92, 99–101
  problems of, 53–55, 90, 92
  property of, 7, 89
  rights of, 6, 32
  role of, 89
  will and testament of, 8
Pattern theory, 63
Peristalsis, 24
Personality, 27–28
Perspiration, 83–84
Phagocytes, 44
Phagocytosis, 48
Pharmacist, 39
Pharmacy, 39
Phenylalanine, 16
Phenylketonuria, 16, 46
Physical handicap, 15
Physicist, 39
Physiology, 21
Physiopathology, 21
Physiotherapist, 32, 33–34, 70
Pituitary gland, 46
Play, 86–87
Poisons, 39, 45, 46, 50, 52
  chemical, 46, 49
  vegetable, 49
Population census, 17
Post-mortem, 61
Pressure sores, 54
  in elderly patients, 4
  treatment of, 104
Primary health care, 18
Professional ethics, 4, 11
Professional misconduct, 5, 6, 40
Prognosis, 47
Projection, 42
Prosthesis, 28
Protoplasm, 21
Psychiatric nurse, 46
Psychiatrists, 46
Psychosomatic illness, 41, 46
Pulse, in the dying, 59
Pyelonephritis, 98

Radiation, 39, 45
Radioactive materials, 39
Radiotherapist, 39
Radiotherapy, 67, 69
Radium, 39
Rationalisation, 42
Reality orientation programme, 41
Receptionist, 34
Recreational activities, 87
Rectum, 84
Reflex action, 25
Registrar, 60, 61
Registrar General, 17
Regression, 28, 41
Relationships, 27, 28, 30
  human, 5
  mother and child, 29

nurse – employer, 9–11
nurse – patient, 2, 6
Relaxation, 75, 86
Religion, 58, 84
  differences in, 59
  Jewish, 59
  minister of, 58
  Muslim, 58, 59, 88
  Roman Catholic, 58
  Romany, 58
Renal system, 84
Report of the Committee on Nursing
  1972, 1
Repression, 42
Reproduction, 26
  bisexual, 26
  by cell division, 26
Reproductive cycle, 26
Research, 2, 3, 4, 5, 51, 54, 63, 87, 103–
  108
  collection of data in, 106
  descriptive, 105
  empirical, 105
  ethics of, 106
  experimental, 105
  feasibility of, 106
  influence on nursing of, 107–108
  non-empirical, 105
  reports of, 107
  survey, 105
Respiration, 23, 82, 83–84
  in the dying, 59
  rate and depth of, 23
  see also Breathing
Respiratory system, 82
Rest, 53
Rheumatoid arthritis, 46, 91
Right to practise, 5
Rites of passage, 89
Roles, 31
  and behaviour, 31
Royal College of Nursing, 5
Royal Society for the Prevention of
  Accidents, 45
Rubella, 15

Safety, 11, 13, 38, 52, 84, 100–101
  physiological, 84
  psychological, 84–85
  social, 85
Salmonella, 50
Sanitation, 16
Sarcoma, 45
Sebaceous glands, 22
Sebum, 22
Secretions, 43
  vaginal, 43
Sensation, 25–26
Sense organs, 25
Sensory nerve endings, 26
Septicaemia, 48
Service, 1
Sexuality, 85, 100
Shelter, 16
Shock, 43
  due to pain, 43
  prolonged, 43
Side-effects, 46
Sight, partial loss of, 54
Signs, 21
Skin, 21, 44
  breakdown of, 92
  care of, 86
  changes in the dying, 59

Slander, 9
Sleep, 53, 87
  deep, 87
  desynchronised, 87
  synchronised, 87
Smoking, 43
  during pregnancy, 29, 33
Social class, 17
Social worker, 32, 33, 36, 70
Spastics, 15
Specificity theory, 63
Spermatozoon, 26
St John Ambulance Brigade, 33
Staphylococci, 50
Sterilisation, 52
Stress, 5, 13, 15, 16, 41, 46, 83
Stroke, 54, 94
Sublimation, 42
Sunburn, 45
Sweat, 25
  insensible, 25
Symptoms, 19, 20, 53
  relief of, 53
Syphilis, 43
System, 21, 22

Tears, 43, 44
Teratoma, 45
Terminal care, 57
Thyroid gland, 23, 46
  failure of development of, 16
Thyroxine, 16, 23
Tissue, 21, 22, 44
  blood supply to, 54
  connective, 45
  epithelial, 45
  lymphoid, 44
  nervous, 45
  rejection of, 62
  skeletal, 45
  transplantation of, 62
  typing of, 62
Tonsils, 44
Toxaemia, 48
Toxins, 48, 50
  attenuated, 48
Toxoid, 48
  diphtheria, 48
  tetanus, 48
Trade Union and Labour Relations Act
  1974, 11
Training, 2, 3–4
  plan of, 10
  professional, 10
  regulations for, 10
  syllabus of, 3
Transplantation, 62
  organs for, 60
Trauma, 45
Tumours, 45
  benign, 45

Ulcer, 54
United Kingdom Central Council, 6
Urine, 25, 43, 83
  pH reaction of, 43
  retention of, 98
  volume and concentration of, 83

Vaccine, 45
  triple, 48
  whooping cough, 48
Varicose veins, 97
Ventilation, 47, 51

Viraemia, 48
Viruses, 47, 48–49, 51
Voluntary agencies, 33

Walking, 53–54
Water
    elimination of, 83
    loss from skin, 25
    need for, 83, 99
Water supply, pure, 16
Will, 8
Work, 86–87
World Health Organization, 13, 16, 18

Zygote, 26